Children and Young People's Nursing Skills
at a Glance

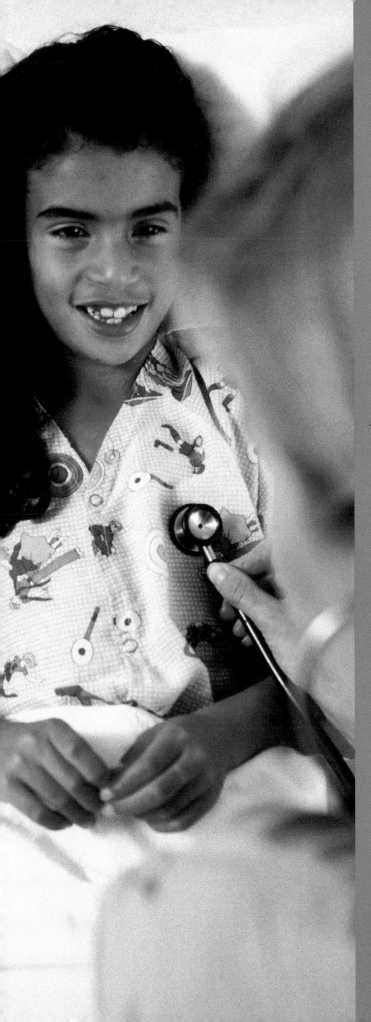

Children and
Young People's
Nursing Skills
at a Glance

Edited by

Elizabeth Gormley-Fleming
Head of Department for Nursing (Children's,
Learning Disability and Mental Health) and
Social Work
School of Health and Social Work
University of Hertfordshire
Hatfield, UK

Deborah Martin
Senior Lecturer Children's Nursing
University of Hertfordshire
Hatfield, UK

Series Editor
Ian Peate

WILEY Blackwell

This edition first published 2018
© 2018 John Wiley & Sons Ltd.

The right of Elizabeth Gormley-Fleming and Deborah Martin to be identified as the authors of the editorial material in this work has been asserted in accordance with law.

Registered Offices   John Wiley & Sons, Inc., 111 River Street, Hoboken, NJ 07030, USA
John Wiley & Sons Ltd, The Atrium, Southern Gate, Chichester,
West Sussex, PO19 8SQ, UK

Editorial Office   9600 Garsington Road, Oxford, OX4 2DQ, UK

For details of our global editorial offices, customer services, and more information about Wiley products visit us at www.wiley.com.

Wiley also publishes its books in a variety of electronic formats and by print-on-demand. Some content that appears in standard print versions of this book may not be available in other formats.

Limit of Liability/Disclaimer of Warranty

Library of Congress Cataloging-in-Publication Data are available

ISBN: 9781119078531

Cover image: © Keith Brofsky/Gettyimages

Set in Minion Pro 9.5/11.5 by Aptara
Printed and bound by CPI Group (UK) Ltd, Croydon, CR0 4YY

10 9 8 7 6 5 4 3 2 1

Contents

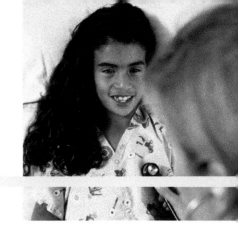

Contributors

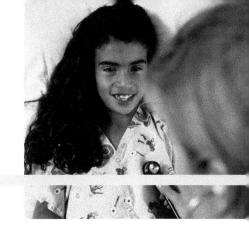

Elizabeth Akers, Chapters 12, 51, 52

Ceri Baker, Chapters 15, 39

Catherine Beadle, Chapter 50

Hannah Chance, Chapter 32

Samia Choudhury, Chapter 57

Sue Collier, Chapter 7, 8

Julie Enright, Chapters 53, 54

Jenni Etchells, Chapters 65, 66

Ericia Everett, Chapter 56

Lynn Fanning, Chapter 24

Liz Gormley-Fleming, Chapters 5, 11, 13, 14, 16, 17, 20, 21, 22, 23, 26, 30, 31, 34, 45, 46, 55, 62, 63

Heather Grant Davey, Chapter 6

Amy Halliday, Chapter 40

Anice Kavathekar, Chapter 29, 58

Sue Llewelyn, Chapters 47, 48

Gary Meager, Chapters 18, 61

Michele O'Grady, Chapters 25, 44

Amanda Parson, Chapters 49, 64

Julia Petty, Chapters 1, 2, 3, 9, 10, 19, 33, 59

Katrina Polfrey, Chapter 4

Sam Pollard, Chapter 11

Sarah Pratley, Chapters 27, 28

Sheila Roberts, Chapters 41, 42, 43

Gemma Tammas, Chapter 38

Maxine Wallis-Redworth, Chapters 35, 36, 37

Yasemin Zerzavatci, Chapter 60

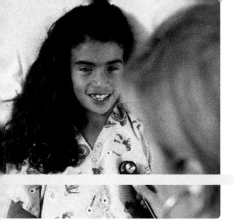

Preface

The prime focus of this text book is to provide evidence-based information in an accessible and easy format for children's and young people's nurses. I hope that the reader will elicit the key points relevant to their practice to enable them to deliver care in a safe and effective manner. The information is delivered in a stimulating visual format along with succinct informative text.

It is not possible to capture the complete set of skills a children's nurse requires in this text book. As with any text book, the contemporary nature of practice is ever changing as new evidence becomes available and the contributors have aimed to keep abreast of this in the creation of this book. The emphasis has been placed on presenting the skills that are fundamental to the learner nurse to acquire during their period of pre-registration education to enable them to achieve competence by the end of their course. The challenge has been to condense the text into a format that identifies the pertinent points and omits unnecessary information. The drawing and photographs have been chosen to illustrate the key points and also to make this text appear interesting to a range of learners.

It must be acknowledged that the continuum of childhood ranges from the neonatal period through to arrival at adulthood, hence the inclusion of the age ranges where required. This is not an exhaustive set of clinical skills in this book pertinent to all within the continuum of childhood as there are other text books in this series such as those that address the neonate and learning disabilities, for example.

The education of nurses is currently undergoing significant changes and the challenge to provide up-to-date education remains constant. This *At a Glance series* will be of interest to current students, health care support workers who work with children and young people, registered nurses who wish to update or consult the literature, and to those future students undertaking associate nurse programmes or those on apprenticeship routes.

This book has been written by experienced practitioners and educators who are all passionate about delivering quality nursing care to the child or young person and their families. Without their contribution, this book would not have been possible, so thank you for contributing and for your time.

Liz Gormley-Fleming

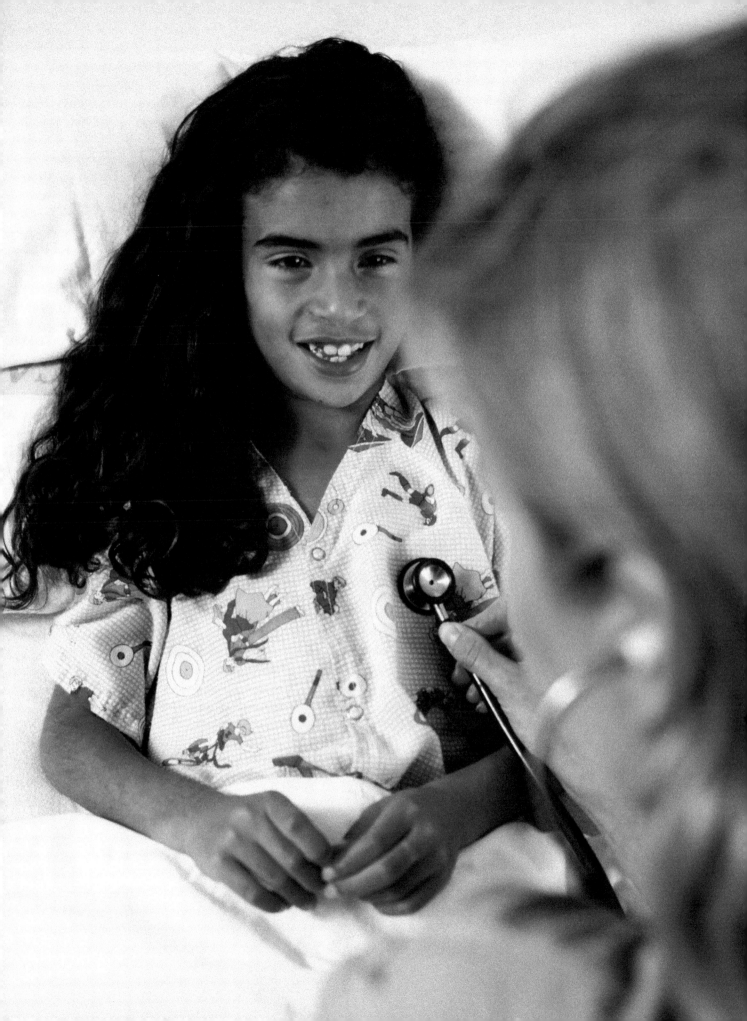

1 Initial assessment: subjective

Subjective assessment of the child's general appearance: Overview

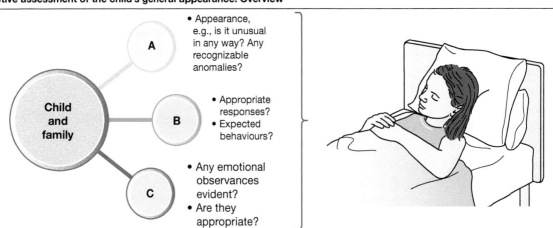

Child and family

A
- Appearance, e.g., is it unusual in any way? Any recognizable anomalies?

B
- Appropriate responses?
- Expected behaviours?

C
- Any emotional observances evident?
- Are they appropriate?

Subjective assessment according to stage of development: Examples

Neonate (0–28 days) and infant (up to 1 year)	Parent–infant interaction. Normal behaviours, reflexes, e.g. rooting, sucking. Expected behaviours, crying, sleeping, consolability Physical signs: body movements, spontaneous, position, symmetry, facial feature
Toddler (1–2 years)	Parent–toddler interaction. Normal behaviours, e.g. separation anxiety, follow simple instructions. Expected developmental milestones, e.g. crawling, walking, early speech
Pre-school / (2–5 years)	Parent–child interaction. Normal behaviours, e.g. able to follow simple instructions Expected developmental milestones, e.g. physical abilities, able to speak/communicate/answer questions
Older child (5–12 years)	Parent–child interaction. Normal behaviours, e.g. greater autonomy Expected developmental milestones, e.g. physical abilities, able to hold a conversation
Adolescent (>12 years)	Parent–teenager interaction. Normal behaviours, e.g. articulation and explanations, social skills. Self-consciousness, body image, state of hygiene

Subjective assessment according to body system: Examples

Respiratory	Presence of audible breathing, cough, wheeze, grunting (babies). Breathing pattern and effort, dyspnoea, shortness of breath, depth and symmetry of breathing efforts, colour – see below
Cardiovascular	What is the colour of the skin, oral mucosa and nail beds? Are these pink? Is there cyanosis present? Or is the skin colour flushed?
Disability: Neurological	Presence of normal or abnormal movements, gait, coordination, and head size and shape? Behavioural responses. Intact senses?
Ear, nose and throat/face	Is a runny nose visible? Is the voice normal or is there huskiness/croakiness/loss of voice? Can the child hear normally? Is the throat red? What is the position of the ears, eyes and facial features? Are there any dysmorphic features?
Fluid balance	Does the child look dehydrated? Sunken eyes, skin colour with reduced turgor, dry, cracked lips, sunked fontanelle (baby)? Is there presence of oedema?
Gastrointestinal	Abdomen size and shape, is there vomiting? Are the weight and size appropriate for age? Is there presence of obesity or failure to thrive? Is the child in pain, holding/guarding their abdomen? Appearance of the umbilicus (baby)
Homeostasis	Does the child feel or look hot/cold? Is there any jitteriness (infant) in the case of a low blood sugar/metabolic disturbances?
Other systems	Appearance may indicate generalized infection. Musculo-skeletal: body/limb proportions, tone, posture, symmetry; is the spine straight or is there any curvature? Skin: nature and distribution of lesions, wounds, bruises, rashes; is there a suspicious appearance?

Children and Young People's Nursing Skills at a Glance, First Edition. Edited by Elizabeth Gormley-Fleming sund Deborah Martin.
© 2018 John Wiley & Sons, Ltd. Published 2018 by John Wiley & Sons, Ltd.

Assessment overview

Assessment is an important component of nursing practice, necessary for the planning and delivery of patient and family-centred care. A comprehensive nursing assessment includes both subjective (qualitative) and objective (quantitative/measurable) elements, namely, general appearance, patient history, physical examination and measurement of vital signs. Of these four components, the area of subjective assessment and observation of clinical appearance is the focus of the present chapter. Objective physical assessment, including history taking and monitoring will follow in subsequent chapters.

Subjective assessment

Subjective nursing assessment is an individualized, qualitative approach that does not use objective, measurements, tools or equipment. Rather, it is based on individualized clinical *observation* relating to the physical, emotional and behavioural characteristics of the child and family. Therefore, by its very nature, such a form of assessment can be open to interpretation and opinion. However, it also serves as an essential starting point to any holistic assessment of a child and family. Inspection and observation of general appearance and behaviour are therefore an integral part of an *initial* assessment before any objective data can be recorded. The skills of performing sound, clinical observation and judgement develop over time and through experience by nursing students and beyond into qualification. The importance of such skills should not be underestimated. It should also be remembered that parents or primary caregivers are best placed to recognize concerns and will report these based on subjective observations of changes in their child's physical or emotional state. This information should be considered alongside nursing assessment data.

How to perform a subjective assessment

The initial nursing assessment of a child should be undertaken with a parent or known caregiver upon arrival to a ward, on pre-admission or, in the case of out-of-hospital care, at the first meeting following introduction to a new child and family in line with any referral for ongoing care. Ideally, initial assessment should be completed within 24 hours of admission and any key information should be documented clearly using appropriate records.

Observation can be carried out while taking the history and establishing rapport. This can be done in conjunction with observations by and from the parents, if present, along with sound clinical nursing judgement. For example, you can observe the child's behaviour, level of understanding and general appearance on admission at first introduction and consider this with the parents' own reports. General appearance of the child and family includes observation of their physical, behavioural and emotional state. At any age, considerations for the subjective assessment of the child or young person include:

- Do they look well or unwell?
- Are they pale, blue or flushed?
- Are they moving, active or lethargic?
- What is the general posture?
- Are they agitated or calm?
- Are they able to respond appropriately to questioning and are they obeying requests? Or are they resistant in their responses and reaction?
- What is the family reaction and perceived emotional state?

Subjective assessment according to age

Care of the child encompasses a wide range of ages from new-born up to the adolescent period. Although some of the principles of assessing children are similar to assessing adults, children are not just small adults, and the approach to assessment and content can be quite different. Moreover, assessment changes in relation to what to observe as children develop and get older so that eventually, in the young person, it is similar to adults. The Figure aims to highlight the important differences to give some general principles and provide an outline of subjective assessment in different age groups. This emphasizes that the approach to subjective assessment is influenced by a child's age, stage of development and level of understanding.

In the neonatal and infant period, physical assessment includes, for example, observation of facial features, symmetry, posture, movement and tone of the limbs. Behavioural elements include presence of a strong cry and normal responses to being held/consoled. Emotional elements include observation of interaction between them and their parents. In the young child, gross physical and fine motor skills can be observed according to age expectations, with refinement occurring as the child gets older. Age-appropriate speech and language can also be noted. Behaviour can be observed by a child's mood and, again, interaction with parents. In an adolescent, similar points can be addressed but in line with behaviours applicable to teenage years, including level and type of communication and emotional reaction.

Subjective assessment according to body system

Subjective assessment can also be carried out according to the biological system, as is commonly used in the systematic approach to holistic physical examination. This will be covered in greater detail in Chapter 3. A full examination of all the systems is the most thorough way to gain a complete physical picture of the child or young person. The subjective components of these systems are displayed in the Figure.

To conclude, sound clinical judgement goes hand in hand with subjective nursing assessment and should be used to make decisions on the need for further, more objective, and possibly more invasive assessment methods.

Key points
- Subjective nursing assessment should include inspection and general observation. These are the important parts of any initial assessment or examination, undertaken in conjunction with the parents or caregivers where possible.
- Subjective assessment should include the physical, behavioural and emotional characteristics of the child or young person and their family.
- The approach to subjective assessment is influenced by the age of the child or young person, their developmental stage and level of understanding.

Further reading

Broom, M. (2007) Exploring the assessment process. *Paediatric Nursing*, **19**(4), 22–25.

Engel, J. K. (2006) *Mosby's Pocket Guide to Pediatric Assessment*, 5th edn. Mosby, New York.

Roland, D., Lewis, G. and Davies, F. (2011) Addition of a subjective nursing assessment improves specificity of a tool to predict admission of children to hospital from an emergency department. *Pediatric Research*, 70, 587.

2 History taking

History taking overview

Taking a patient history includes

✓ Establishing a rapport with the patient and his or her family

✓ Using effective communication skills. See communication framework figure

✓ Gathering information on:
  ✓ the current concern, using both open and closed questions

✓ SAMPLE (see below) may be useful as a prompt, to include;
  ✓ symptoms experienced
  ✓ medical history, and medication
  ✓ the patient's overall health status
  ✓ family and social
  ✓ perception of his or her well-being

✓ Asking about emotional health

✓ Discover the family's perspective

✓ Closure, with rapport maintained

✓ Documenting clearly and thoroughly

Communication framework for history taking
Source: Adapted from Kurtz et al., 1998

Calgary-Cambridge framework for effective communication – adapted for children

1. Initiating the session
Establish initial rapport with child and family

2. Gathering information
Explore the patient's problem
Understand the patient's perspective

3. Building the relationship
Develop rapport. Involve the child and family

4. Providing structure to the interview
Summarizing, signposting. Sequencing, timing

5. Explanation and planning
Provide the correct amount and type of information
Aid accurate recall and understanding
Achieve a shared understanding

6. Close the session

Using SAMPLE to obtain a child's health history

S Symptoms What symptoms are experienced and how have they developed? How have they been managed?

A Allergies Are there any known allergies? Has there been a reaction to something leading to the symptoms?

M Medications Is the child taking any medications, either prescribed or other?

P Past history Have there been any previous medical, psychological, or social conditions/illnesses?

L Last eaten and drank? When did the child last have anything to eat or drink?

E Events What events occurred that led to the current situation? E.g. external events such as accidents

Examples of questions to obtain a child's health history: according to the systems

☐ Airway and breathing – Has the child had problems with their breathing?
☐ Cardiovascular – Does the child's skin change colour when crying? If so, what colour do you see?
☐ Disability (neurological) – Does the child tire easily or sleep excessively?
☐ ENT – Does the child frequently develop streptococcal pharyngitis (strep throat)?
☐ Fluids – Is the child passing urine? Drinking?
☐ Gastrointestinal – Does the child have feeding difficulty?
☐ Homeostasis – Has the child been feverish?
☐ Skin – Is the child showing a rash or other skin sign?
☐ Musculo-skeletal – Does the child have any problems with activity and co-ordination?aaaa

Examples of questions to obtain a child's medical and nursing health history: according to age

☐ Are there any delays or recent concerns with expected developmental and age-appropriate milestones – physical,/motor, behavioural, corgitive?
☐ Has the child experienced any growth delay, weight loss or increase?
☐ Are there any age-specific issues to consider, e.g. in babies, were there any antenatal issues of note? What is the pattern of bowel movements, number of wet nappies, sleeping and waking for feeds? In the older child, are there any changes to their activity levels, reports of pain and discomfort, exposure to infections at nursery/school?

Children and Young People's Nursing Skills at a Glance, First Edition. Edited by Elizabeth Gormley-Fleming and Deborah Martin.
© 2018 John Wiley & Sons, Ltd. Published 2018 by John Wiley & Sons, Ltd.

History taking overview

History taking is a key component of a nursing patient assessment and an important part of prioritizing and planning care. Traditionally, a medical history is undertaken for a diagnosis and to ultimately decide on appropriate treatment. A nursing history should be carried out jointly and is regarded as a key skill that develops through experience. It should include physical, social and psycho-emotional domains. In its simplest form, history taking involves asking appropriate questions to children, young people and/or their families to obtain vital information to assist the subsequent care. An overview of history taking and its components can be seen in the Figure.

The aims of history taking can be summarized as:

• to find out more about presenting symptoms and identify problems that may not be immediately obvious;
• to direct necessary examination and further investigations;
• to reach a definite or differential diagnosis;
• to establish a rapport and a therapeutic relationship with the child and parents;
• to tailor appropriate treatment strategies.

Nursing history taking fits well with a person-centred approach to care where nurses are expected to get to know their patients and understand the needs and problems of the children in their care. Integral to this process is the need for effective communication skills, which should aim to achieve holistic, thorough history taking in the context of a therapeutic relationship.

Communication skills in history taking

An essential part of person-centred communication during history taking is the establishment of rapport between the nurse and child or young person and family. See the Figure for the Calgary-Cambridge communication framework that can be used to understand the vital elements of this process. This covers elements that are required for any patient but they can easily be applied to a child, young person and their parents.

Other factors need to be considered in relation to communication during history taking. If a child or family does not speak English, it will be necessary to arrange an interpreter to clarify what is said. In addition, for very young children or those who have no or limited speech, the history is taken from the parents. In older children, there must be a balance between giving them independence and getting a full account of the illness or situation.

Communication during history taking may also be compromised by factors such as the child's distress. Parents may be extremely anxious, particularly in settings such as accident and emergency rooms. Histories may therefore need to be brief and focused. If a comprehensive history is not achievable in the first instance, it may be necessary to continue adding detail later. The nature of nursing means that relationships between nurses and children or young people in their care can be developed over a longer period, with more frequent contact than other members of the multi-disciplinary team. Within this context, history taking can be seen as a process of getting to know the child and family better and to understand their needs and concerns. It can also be viewed as an incremental process where information is accumulated over time. This means history taking need not necessarily take place in a formal consultation and can take place informally, depending on the situation. Whatever mode is employed, there are key components of any history taking, discussed below.

The history-taking process

In the hospital setting, history taking can follow a structured approach using, for example, a mnemonic to aid comprehensive information gathering. One example of such a framework is the mnemonic SAMPLE.

S = *symptoms* in relation to the current concern or presenting complaint. For example; when and how did the symptoms start? Was the child well before? Have there been similar episodes or similar illnesses in the family or school?
A = *allergies* and whether the child has any existing reaction to a known substance.
M = *medication.* Is the child currently taking any prescribed drugs? In addition, if recreational drug use is a possibility, this can also be considered here.
P = *past medical history of the child* which is a key element in history taking. This can look back as far as pregnancy. For example, in babies, were any factors relevant to foetal development and well-being important such as antenatal infection, blood group incompatibility, maternal illness? What was the gestation and birth weight? Were there any birth injuries or the need for resuscitation? In children, have there been any previous illnesses or are there any systems that require particular attention. A developmental approach can also be considered as well as the social, mental and family history.
L = when did the child *last eat and drink*?
E = whether there were any *events* that led to the current situation, for example, accidents?

Finally, it is essential that a compassionate approach be upheld in history taking which demonstrates attention to privacy and dignity as well as upholding confidentiality. This may not be easy in a busy environment where space is limited. This highlights the potential ethico-legal implications in relation to how information is collected and protected. Additionally, issues of safeguarding are also important to take account of recognizing that not all parents or carers have the child's best interests at heart and may conceal vital facts, hindering a full and accurate picture. Multi-disciplinary support in such cases may be sought.

Key points

• History taking is an integral component of holistic assessment to be considered in line with subjective assessment and objective measurements.
• History taking is a process of asking appropriate questions in order to gather information and gain a comprehensive picture of the child's presenting problem.
• History taking in children and young people should be done in collaboration with parent reports, where possible, having established a sound rapport to aid effective communication and to start the therapeutic process.

Further reading

Fawcett, T. and Rhynas, S. (2012) Taking a patient history: the role of a nurse. *Nursing Standard*, **26**(24), 41–46.
Kurtz, S. M., Silverman, J. and Draper, J. (2005) *Teaching and Learning Communication Skills in Medicine.* Radcliffe Medical Press, Oxford.
McKenna, L., Innes, K., French, J., Streitberg, S. and Gilmour, C. (2010) Is history taking a dying skill? An exploration using a simulated learning environment. *Nurse Education in Practice*, **11**(4), 234–238.

③ Principles of systematic assessment

Source: Adapted from Resuscitation Council (UK) (2014) Guidelines and guidance: The ABCDE approach. https://www.resus.org.uk/resuscitation-guidelines/abcde-approach

Summary points of the ABCDE approach

Airway, Breathing, Circulation, Disability, Exposure

⬇

Universal principles for all children and young people

⬇

Apply when critical illness or injury is suspected or evident

⬇

Assess and treat continuously and simultaneously

⬇

Treat life-threatening signs immediately

⬇

Life-saving treatment does not require a definitive diagnosis

⬇

Reassess regularly and at any sign of deterioration

Primary – secondary – tertiary assessment

1 — The initial assessment and systemic approach to checking for life-threatening problems – ABCDE

2 — A more detailed examination and focused history

3 — Further investigations to aid diagnosis following stabilization

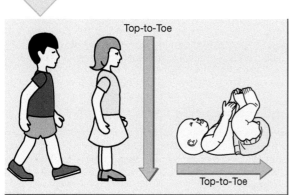

Top-to-Toe

A systematic Top-to-Toe approach to physical assessment in an infant

Source: Adapted from GOV UK Newborn and infant physical examination: clinical guidance. https://www.gov.uk/government/collections/newborn-and-infant-physical-examination-clinical-guidance)

- Appearance, including colour, breathing, behaviour, activity and posture
- Head (including fontanelles), face, nose, mouth including palate, ears, neck and general symmetry of head and facial features. Note head circumference
- Eyes: check opacities and 'red reflex'
- Neck and clavicles, limbs hand, feet and digits: assess proportions and symmetry
- Heart: check position, rate, rhythm and sounds, murmurs and femoral pulse volume
- Lungs: check effort, rate and sounds
- Abdomen: check shape and palpate to identify any organomegaly, umbilical cord
- Genitalia and anus: check completeness and patency and undescended testes in males
- Spine: palpate bony structures and check skin
- Skin: note colour and texture, birthmarks or rashes
- Central nervous system: check tone, behaviour, movements and posture, and elicit reflexes only if concerned
- Hips: check symmetry of limbs and skin folds; perform Barlow and Ortolani's manoeuvres
- Cry: note sound
- Weight: note

The ABCDE approach Source: Adapted from Resuscitation Council (UK) (2014) Guidelines and guidance: The ABCDE approach https://www.resus.org.uk/resuscitation-guidelines/abcde-approach

	Assessment
A – Airway	Airway clear? Voice Breath sounds
B – Breathing	Respiratory rate Chest wall movement Chest percussion Lung auscultation Pulse oximetry
C – Circulation	Skin colour, sweating Capillary refill time Palpate pulse rate Heart auscultation Blood pressure Electrocardiography monitoring
D – Disability	Level of consciousness and neurological status AVPU • Alert • Voice responsive • Pain responsive • Unresponsive Limb movements Pupillary light reflexes Blood glucose
E – Exposure	Exposed skin Temperature

Systematic assessment overview

Assessment of the child or young person and family is multi-faceted. The important components include subjective observation and history taking, as discussed in Chapters 1 and 2, along with objective measurements and monitoring data, depending on the individual situation. In order to manage the assessment process and ensure vital- elements are not missed, it is useful to employ a systematic approach to assessment that can guide the nurse through the process with a logical structure.

The ABCDE approach

The well-documented and recommended approach to systematic assessment is the ABCDE approach: **A**irway, **B**reathing, **C**irculation, **D**isability (Neurological), **E**xposure. Such a mnemonic-based approach has previously been highlighted by the use of SAMPLE for history taking (see Chapter 2) serving to guide assessment in a structured and logical way. The ABCDE mnemonic is endorsed by Resuscitation Councils worldwide. However, this approach does not just apply to resuscitation; it also applies to the context of emergency care or critical illness or injury as highlighted in the Figure.

The ABCDE approach is applicable in all clinical emergencies. It can be used in the street without any equipment or, in a more advanced form, upon the arrival of the emergency medical services, in emergency rooms, in general wards of hospitals, or in intensive care units. Each stage of the ABCDE approach is outlined in detail in the Figure.

The aims of the ABCDE approach are:

• to provide life-saving treatment;
• to break down complex clinical situations into more manageable parts;
• to serve as an assessment and treatment algorithm;
• to establish common situational awareness among all health professionals.

The ABCDE approach is applicable to all patients, both adults and children. The clinical signs of critical conditions are similar, regardless of the underlying cause. This makes exact knowledge of the underlying cause unnecessary when performing the initial assessment and treatment. The ABCDE approach should be used whenever critical illness or injury is suspected. It is a valuable tool for identifying or ruling out critical conditions in daily practice. Respiratory or cardiac arrest is often preceded by adverse clinical signs and these can be recognized by applying the ABCDE approach to potentially prevent this situation. ABCDE is also recommended as the first step in post-resuscitation care upon the return of spontaneous breathing and circulation.

It is important that the order from A through to E is maintained. For example, there is no point addressing circulation if the airway is not patent. In addition, regular reassessment is essential after each stage and remains the case in any event where a child deteriorates. The ABCDE approach and the importance of reassessment will be emphasized again in Chapters 56–59.

Primary – secondary – tertiary assessment

Systematic assessment can also be considered in relation to three phases: primary, secondary, and tertiary. ABCDE is part of primary assessment along with subjective observation (see Chapter 1). Once this has been undertaken and reassessment has confirmed a desired outcome (i.e. the situation is no longer life-threatening), then one can move to secondary assessment. This is a more thorough examination and focused history of the child or young person. History taking is covered in Chapter 2. Finally, further assessment by investigations and monitoring are part of the tertiary phase.

Systematic physical assessment

A structured approach to assessment can use the systems of the body in relation to the physical examination of a child. Such a method is used, for example, to examine newborn babies at discharge from hospital and neonates at their six-week postnatal check. A head-to-toe approach works through each of the systems. Conducting a head-to-toe assessment ensures that a nurse is thorough in the assessment of the child. By starting at the head and working down to the feet, this ensures that nothing is missed in any of the major body systems. This type of assessment means that a nurse is checking all systems for abnormalities and is less likely to miss any problems. The head-to-toe assessment follows a logical sequence starting at the head and neck, moves on to the chest, then to the abdomen and limbs.

Assessment tools for a systematic approach

In nursing practice, a systematic approach to assessment can be aided by the use of assessment tools. Mnemonics such as SAMPLE and ABCDE are tools in that they serve to guide practice logically in order to ensure a thorough assessment. Examples of other assessment tools are:

• AVPU (**A**lert – **V**oice – **P**ain – **U**nresponsive): Measure the level of neurological response as part of the **D** (Disability / neurological) component of ABCDE: see later chapters.
• Pain assessment tools: the presence of pain is assessed on a number of criteria comprising physiological, behavioural and biochemical signs. The score indicates the level of pain and guides appropriate analgesia. On a more simplistic level, pain can be assessed by asking a child to grade their pain from a selection of graded scores.
• PEWS (**P**aediatric **E**arly **W**arning **S**core): see later chapters.
• GCS (**G**lasgow **C**oma **S**cale); see later chapters.
• Skin assessment tools (e.g. Braden Q and Glamorgan tools: see Chapter 19). Skin is assessed on a range of criteria, each one scored on a scale of 1–4 with the total score indicative of the risk of skin breakdown.

Key points

• Assessment of the sick or injured child can be facilitated by a systematic approach, which gives a logical structure and avoids omissions.
• The ABCDE framework is a well-documented and widely used systematic approach to assessment; an integral component of primary assessment.
• Systematic assessment can be further assisted by the use of tools, which serve to guide assessment.

References

GOV.UK (2014) Newborn and infant physical examination: clinical guidance. Available at: https://www.gov.uk/government/collections/newborn-and-infant-physical-examination-clinical-guidance
Resuscitation Council (UK) (2014) *Guidelines and Guidance: The ABCDE Approach*. Available at: https://www.resuscitation-guidelines.org.uk/resuscitation-guidelines/abcde-approach/

Further reading

Dieckmann, R. A., Brownstein, D. and Gausche-Hill, M. (2010) The pediatric assessment triangle: a novel approach for the rapid evaluation of children. *Pediatric Emergency Care*, **26**(4), 312–315.
Jevon, P. (2012) *Paediatric Advanced Life Support: A Practical Guide for Nurses*, 2nd edn. Blackwell, Oxford.
NHS Institute for Innovation and Improvement (2013) PEWS charts. Available at: http://www.institute.nhs.uk/safer_care/paediatric_safer_care/pews_charts.html

4 Communication

Types of communication

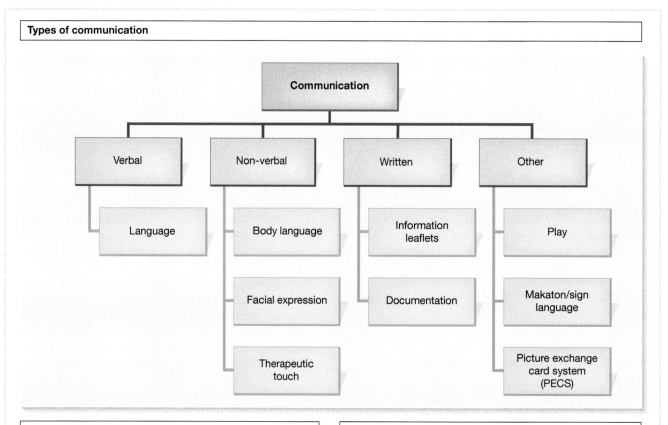

Communication

- **Verbal**
  - Language
- **Non-verbal**
  - Body language
  - Facial expression
  - Therapeutic touch
- **Written**
  - Information leaflets
  - Documentation
- **Other**
  - Play
  - Makaton/sign language
  - Picture exchange card system (PECS)

Play during the assessment process

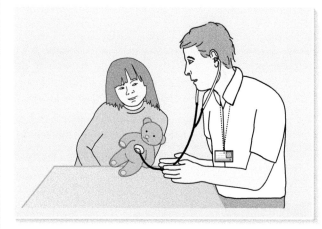

Barriers to effective communication

- Cognitive ability/disability
- Individual understanding
- Language
- Culture
- Emotion
- Distractions
- Environment

Improving communication

Technique to improve communication

- Where possible, create a quiet, comfortable environment
- Adopt an open posture, be aware of your own body language
- Introduce yourself to the child and family
- Explain the assessment process
- Maintain eye contact
- Allow time for the child/parent/carer to answer questions
- Use active listening skills
- Use age-appropriate techniques/language
- Facilitate play, as appropriate to the child's age
- Avoid the use of jargon
- Facilitate therapeutic relationships with both the child and family, building trust will increase communication

Children and Young People's Nursing Skills at a Glance, First Edition. Edited by Elizabeth Gormley-Fleming and Deborah Martin.
© 2018 John Wiley & Sons, Ltd. Published 2018 by John Wiley & Sons, Ltd.

Communication overview

Communication is an essential skill in the assessment and care of children, young people and their families. There are four main types of communication, each with sub-areas to aid the sharing and understanding of information.

Types of communication

Verbal

When communicating verbally, the type of language used should be considered, avoiding the use of jargon. For children and families whose first language is not English, interpreting services should be used, ensuring individual needs are met. The ability to understand, on the part of both child and family, should be considered, taking into account age, developmental level and cognitive ability, adapting the language and approach used as necessary.

Non-verbal

Non-verbal communication techniques, such as active listening, body language, facial expressions and therapeutic touch, contribute to a large portion of how information is conveyed and received. Active listening skills require the listener to make a conscious effort to focus on what is being said, improving their ability to understand information. Body language, such as eye contact, sitting directly opposite, nodding and an open posture, also demonstrate that the listener is interested and engaged in the conversation, encouraging the speaker to continue with the sharing of information; essential during the assessment process.

Written

In relation to assessment, documentation is essential, acting as a record of the information obtained from the child and family. It also enables the sharing of information between professionals within the multi-disciplinary team. When documenting information, all records should be factual and accurate, with a date, time and signature on completion.

Play

To accurately assess a child it is necessary to build a therapeutic relationship with the child, gaining their trust and reducing anxiety; all of which increase the accuracy of assessment. A central technique to this is the use of play. Play can be used to do the following:

• Distract during the assessment process, particularly when assessing vital signs.
• Decrease the child's anxiety and consequently reduce the parent's stress.
• Demonstrate the assessment process to the child, aiding their ability to understand and reducing anxiety.
• Promote the hospital environment as a friendly environment to the child, increasing their trust.

When considering the use of play, age-appropriate toys should be used, considering the child's developmental stage. It may also be useful to ask the child's parents/carers what type of toys/activities the child enjoys, increasing the ability to interact and engage with the child.

Makaton/sign language/PECS

All children should be provided with the tools and ability to communicate in the most appropriate way based on their individual ability. It may therefore be necessary to consider the use of alternative methods such as Makaton, sign language and the Picture Exchange Card System (PECS) to ensure that all children and families are provided with the tools to effectively communicate with healthcare professionals.

Improving communication

Although communication is essential to accurate assessment, there are numerous barriers that impact on the effectiveness of communication, negatively impacting the assessment process. Techniques to improve communication should therefore be consider and used, improving the ability to effectively interact with the child and their family, facilitating the building of therapeutic relationship, gaining trust and increasing the ability to accurately assess and care for children/young people and their families.

Key points
• Good communication is essential for the delivery of safe and effective care.
• A range of communications skills is required.
• The foundation for excellent nursing care is communication.

5 Developmental considerations

Growth and development begin at birth. Development referes to an increase in capability of function. Infants and children pass through predictable stages of development

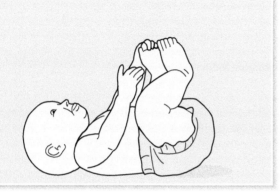

Development is an important indicator of the overall well-being of a child. Assessment of the developmental milestones is an integral part of all nursing and medical assessment of the child

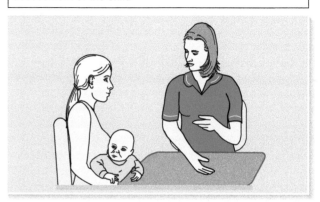

Four areas of development

- Gross motor
- Fine motor
- Social development
- Speech and language development

Hearing and vision need consideration also.

When assessing developmental milestones

- Observe the child informally: young children may not co-operate with you

- Listen to the parents: parental reporting of skills may be all you will get as the child may not want to talk to you

- Prepare your environment: distraction will not be helpful

- One task at time: young children have short attention spans

- Be succinct in your assessment: know what you are assessing

- Ask for the birth history: correct for prematurity until child is 2 years old

Developmental alert

As development is sequential and predictable, signs of development delay must be identified early. Reassurance that normal development will occur is not appropriate.

Referral to a paediatrician should always be made if any of the following are present:

- Maternal concerns at any age
- Regression of a previously acquired skill
- Failure to smile by the age of 10 weeks
- Hand preference, persistent primitive reflexes, squinting or no display of interest in people, toys, or noise at the age of 6 months
- Not sitting up, no pincer grasp or not saying double-syllable words such as ba-ba, ga-ga at the age of 10 months
- Not able to say ma-ma, da da (specific) by the age of 14 months
- No independent walking, drooling and persistent mouthing and has less than six words at the age of 18 months
- Unresponsive to name
- Not stair climbing by age of 2 years
- Not able to combine two and three words by the age of $2\frac{1}{2}$ (e.g. me outside, more milk)
- Unintelligible speech at the age of 4 years

Children and Young People's Nursing Skills at a Glance, First Edition. Edited by Elizabeth Gormley-Fleming and Deborah Martin.
© 2018 John Wiley & Sons, Ltd. Published 2018 by John Wiley & Sons, Ltd.

Developmental considerations overview

The important developmental considerations are shown below.

Age	Gross motor	Fine motor	Language	Social
Birth	Reflexive Flexed posture Complete head lag Hand fisted		Recognizes parental voice Makes throaty noises	Shows interaction with people's faces Gains satisfaction from being fed, held, rocked, cuddled
One month–six weeks	Head control developing, raises head slightly from prone, pelvis flatter when in prone position. Curved back when sitting, needing adult support.	Shows eye coordination-eyes follow and focus vertically and horizontally	Alert to sound	Smiles responsively
4 months	Lifts head and shoulders when prone. Supports weight on wrists and shifts weight to forearms when prone. No head lag. Intentional rolling over.	Holds a rattle and shakes it purposefully. Brings objects to mouth.	Vocalizes. Coos.	Laughs out loud. Begins to respond to no, no Enjoys sitting up More interested in mother. Enjoys attention and can get bored if alone.
6 months	Arms extend supporting chest off surface when prone Sits with self-propping Stands with support Rolls over well	Reaches for objects and can transfer from hand to hand. Whole hand grasp.	Says 'Ma', 'Da'	
7–8 months	Bounces and bears some weight when standing. May begin some form of mobility	Finger feeds	Makes talking sound in response to others Double babble –'ma ma, da da'	Self-contained play Fear of strangers Eye-to-eye contact when talking
9 months	Gets into sitting position alone	Immature pincer grasp		Enjoys peek-a-boo, waves bye-bye
10–12 months	Pulls to standing and stands holding on Cruises around furniture Stands and walks with one hand	Mature pincer grasp Turns pages in a book Will hand a block/object to an adult Can put balls in a box	Begins to put two words together	Points to get what they want Responds to music Shows fear, anger, affection, jealousy, anxiety and sympathy Increased attention span
12–18 months	Walks independently Stoops down to pick up objects	Can build a tower of three or four blocks by the age of 18 months	Has 10 words of meaning Imitates words Points to objects named by adult	Drinks from a cup Spoon feeding self Imitates adult behaviour Follows directions and requests
18–24 months	Walks up and down stairs Steady gait Kicks a ball in front of them Rides a tricycle with walking action	Scribbles with a pencil Opens door handles Builds a tower of 4–6 blocks	Able to link words together to make short sentences Has 200–300 words Refers to self by pronoun	Imitates parents in domestic activities Likes doll and ball games Enjoys playing with other children Short attention span Spoon-feeds self
2–3 years	Throws objects overhead Pedals tricycle Walks backwards Jumps	Draws a circle Drinks from a straw Can string large beads	900-word vocabulary Talks incessantly Can repeat three numbers	Undresses/dresses themselves except for buttons Feeds themselves Toilet trained by day
4 years	Continuous movement going up and down stairs Climbs well	Draws a cross Attempts to write letters	1,500 words, some number concept and asks many questions	Buttons clothes, laces shoes Imagination active
5 years	Good motor control, climbs and jumps well	Draws a triangle and square Prints first name	2,100-word vocabulary. Talks constantly	Understands friendships Power of reasoning

Key points

- Development is not linear and each child is different.
- The first five years are fundamentally important.
- Parental concerns about developmental delays must be taken seriously.

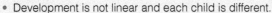

6 Informed consent

Consent should be informed

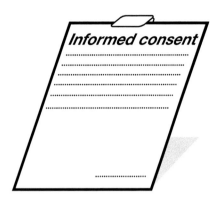

Good communication with the child and parents is essential to gain informed consent

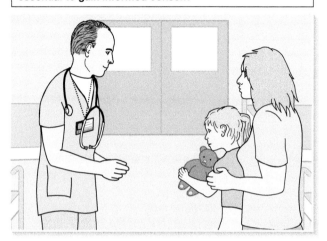

Children can assent to treatment

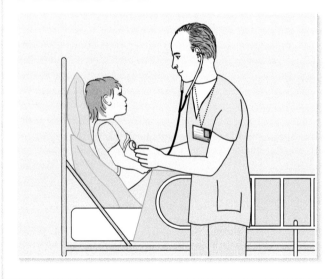

Children and Young People's Nursing Skills at a Glance, First Edition. Edited by Elizabeth Gormley-Fleming and Deborah Martin.
© 2018 John Wiley & Sons, Ltd. Published 2018 by John Wiley & Sons, Ltd.

Informed consent overview

Consent is the principle that a person must give permission before any treatment or examination can be instigated. Valid consent must be sought before the delivery of any aspect of treatment or care. The child or young person and their parents or legal carers should be fully informed and be given sufficient time to consider the information they have been received, along with the opportunity to ask any questions before any care is carried out. The child's developing cognitive ability must be considered, this recognizes the rights of the child in self-determination.

Verbal, written and implied consent

Consent can be gained verbally, can be written or it can be implied. Verbal consent involves asking the child if they are happy to go ahead with treatment or care. This is usually used for less risky treatments and many day-to-day treatments and tests, for example, recording of vital signs.

Written consent is evidence that the child and parents/carers agree to the proposed treatment following the sharing of information. The consent form also requires the signature of the health professional who has appropriate knowledge of the procedure to be undertaken. This must be in accordance with local policy. Written consent is especially important when treatment carries risk, is lengthy or complex.

Implied consent is used in situations where the child makes it clear that they are giving consent. For example; the child pulls their sleeve up when asked if they will have their blood pressure recorded. The nurse should always tell the patient what she intends to do to avoid misinterpretation.

Informed consent and capacity

In order for consent to be informed, the child (in line with Fraser guidelines) and their parents/carers must be in receipt of the correct information. This includes being made aware of the risks and likely effects of the treatment. This information should be delivered in an age-appropriate language. Evaluating competency to give consent is an important part of the process. Children's competence is not determined by their chronological age but by their maturity and understanding. Capacity should always be assessed when gaining consent. Competence is decision-specific and should be considered only in relation to the decision that needs to be made at that time. The test of competence that can be applied involves the child doing the following:

- understanding the treatment required;
- comprehending the implications of any such treatment effects and side effects/risks;
- retaining the information for long enough to make an informed decision;
- giving their consent freely.

The Mental Capacity Act, 2005, describes a person who lacks capacity as someone, therefore, who is unable to make a decision for themselves because of an impairment or disturbance in the functioning of their mind or brain. This can involve disability, a condition, trauma or the effects of drugs or alcohol.

Consent in under-16–18-year-olds

Between the ages of 16 and 17 years, young people are permitted to consent to treatment under the Family Law Reform Act (1969). However, if they refuse to consent to treatment of a mental health issue, they cannot be admitted to hospital on the basis of consent given by someone with parental responsibility. They can be detained under the Mental Health Act of 1983.

Parental responsibility

A person with parental responsibility for a child could be: the child's mother, the biological father, the legal guardian, a person with a residence order concerning the child, a local authority designated to care for the child, or a person with an emergency protection order for the child. If one parent with parental responsibility agrees and the other does not, the health professional will decide if the treatment will proceed or not. If there is disagreement, then legal advice will need to be sought.

When consent is not necessary

There are a few exceptions where treatment can go ahead without consent. For example; if treatment is required in an emergency situation and the child is unable to give consent, or during an operation if the immediate need of an additional procedure to treat a life-threatening problem arises, or in the presence of severe mental health conditions and capacity to consent is diminished.

In the case of major trauma where the child may be unconscious, they may receive treatments that are essential to preserve life. In law, this is permitted as it is in the best interests of the patient.

Key points
- Children have the right to make informed decisions about their care and treatment.
- Children can consent to treatment if professionals feel they are competent to do so, but they cannot refuse treatment.
- All children and parents/carers should be asked for their consent before starting any form of treatment/care.
- In an emergency, treatment may be given without consent.
- The refusal of treatment by either the child and/or parents may be overruled if it is decided that it is in the child's best interest to receive treatment. Legal advice will be sought.

Further reading

Department of Health (2009) *Reference Guide to Consent for Examination or Treatment*, 2nd edn. Department of Health, London.

7 Safeguarding

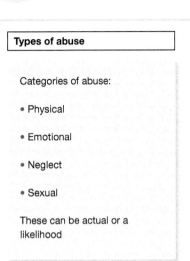

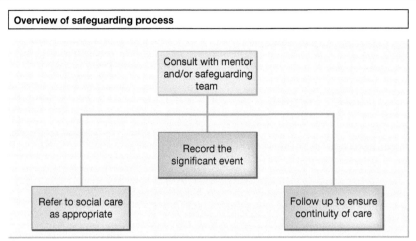

Types of abuse

Categories of abuse:

- Physical

- Emotional

- Neglect

- Sexual

These can be actual or a likelihood

Overview of safeguarding process

Consult with mentor and/or safeguarding team

Record the significant event

Refer to social care as appropriate

Follow up to ensure continuity of care

Child or young person predictive factors

- Pre-term birth

- Born sick

- Chronic illness

- Physical disability

- Learning disability

- Born unwanted

- Born following difficult labour or delivery

- Difficulty with feeding

- Children looked after (in care, institutional abuse)

Parental predictive factors

- Learning difficulties
- Unhappy childhood
- Poor role models
- Psychological issues
- Mental health issues
- Drug or alcohol misuse
- Chronic illness
- Disability
- Domestic abuse

- Poor relationship history
- Unemployment
- Financial burden
- Frustration
- Poverty
- Social isolation
- Homelessness
- Young parents
- Unsupported parents

Assessment framework
Source: Working Together to Safeguard Children: A guide to inter-agency Working to Safeguard and promote the Welfare of Children. March 2013 http://www.nationalarchives.gov.uk/doc/open-government-licence/version/3/Accessed January 2017

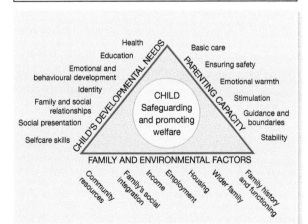

Key points from the Children Act (1998)

Section 17: Provision of services for children in need. These children are defined as:

- Vulnerable children who are unlikely to reach or maintain a satisfactory level of health
- Children whose health or development is likely to be significantly impaired, or further impaired, without help
- Children who are disabled

Section 47: Local Authority's duty to investigate children in need of protection. This duty comes into play in cases when:

- The 'ill treatment or impairment of the health or development of a child... is serious, considerable, noteworthy or important'
- The concept of 'significant harm' is the threshold that justifies compulsory intervention in family life in the best interests of the child

Children and Young People's Nursing Skills at a Glance, First Edition. Edited by Elizabeth Gormley-Fleming and Deborah Martin.
© 2018 John Wiley & Sons, Ltd. Published 2018 by John Wiley & Sons, Ltd.

Safeguarding policy drivers

Safeguarding children and young people is the concern to all members of society. It is everyone's responsibility. Following a high-profile inquiry and serious case review, safeguarding guidance and systems were reviewed. This resulted in a range of new policy guidance being implemented.

The United Nations Convention on the Rights of the Child (UNCRC, 1989) was ratified by the United Kingdom (UK) in 1991. This provides key statements related to provision for children, protection of children and participation in matters which concern them, in a variety of ways, during their childhood.

The commitment of the UK government to the principles of the UNCRC has provided a range of legislation, guidance, strategies and systems to support all professionals to protect children from harm including the Children Act, *Working Together to Safeguard Children* (Department of Education, 2015) and the Munro Reviews of Child Protection practice and services (Department of Education, 2011). Two significant government roles were created; the Children's Minister who represents children and young people at the highest level of government within the Cabinet, and a Children's Commissioner, who listens to children, provides them with information and advises government officials. The UK has four Children's Commissioners.

Following a review of the role of the Children's Commissioner for England, there has been a change from outcomes-based working to a rights-based working.

Care, competence and engagement

Team working is an essential component of children's nursing, however, working in partnership with the inter-professional team and across agencies may result in the formation of transient teams, coming together for the purpose of safeguarding a particular child or young person. This inter-professional and multi-agency working requires a concerted approach. Child abuse and neglect are complex. Children's nurses are required to have a working knowledge of the types of abuse, the policy drivers, the safeguarding process, a working knowledge of mechanisms and systems for safeguarding children and young people in the organization. Achieving continuity of care requires accurate assessment of needs and the risks pertinent to the child or young person, which take into account the growth and developmental milestones, relationships within the family and the environment in which they are being cared for.

Communication and compassion

Effective communication is imperative in information sharing, enabling collaborative working and to plan the resources required to safeguard a child or young person. Children's nurses need to develop skills in working with families and listening to children. This includes developing a trusting and supportive partnership with the family.

The 'best interest' of the child or young person is paramount. Promoting the welfare of the child or young person requires respect for the child or young person. This includes the unborn child. When making disclosures of alleged abuse, children and young people often 'select' a person they feel comfortable to share the information with. In this situation it is important to remain calm, be empathetic, listen carefully to the information, reassure the child or young person and ensure their safety. It is equally important to factually observe and record what you see. An example of this may be that the child or young person is not responding to one of the parents.

Confidentiality in safeguarding is crucial and should be on a 'need-to-know' basis. Information-sharing guidance must be adhered to.

In situations of disclosure, it is important not to prevent a child or young person from freely recalling the significant event. It is important not to ask leading or closed questions or probe for more details. It is vital that evidence is left undisturbed and children and young people are not made promises of secrecy. Be honest with children and young people that the information will need to be shared with a limited range of people to keep them safe. Throughout the whole process, it is crucial to be non-judgemental. Children's nurses have a role in identifying children who are in need, or in need of protection. It is the role of the police and social workers to undertake the investigations.

Courage

Children's nurses have a responsibility to protect the children in their care. They are professionally accountable and responsible for their actions and omissions. The importance of information sharing is key in determining the plan of care for the child and family. Developing professional discernment in this area occurs through experience of safeguarding children and young people. This requires confidence to take action and escalate to key professionals, organizational systems and other agencies. This also requires education and training.

Children's nurses require courage to speak up about any concerns they may have to safeguard a child or young person or to be an advocate for them. Having the courage to ask the seemingly naïve or challenging questions can clarify or explain information that is not understood or partially understood. In addition, professionals in different agencies may not fully understand the intricacies of each other's roles. Assertiveness can avert the need for a serious case review.

Familiarity with the Children Act 1989 is essential for safe practice for all healthcare staff who work with children and young people.

Key points

- Safeguarding children and young people is the responsibility of everyone who comes into contact with them.
- Effective inter-professional and multi-agency working is crucial in safeguarding children and young people.
- Effective communication and record keeping are imperative to safeguard children and young people.
- Working in transient inter-professional teams poses challenges to working together and achieving best practice.
- Have the courage to ask the naïve or challenging questions.
- All healthcare staff must undergo the appropriate level of training.

References

Department of Education (2011) *The Munro Reviews of Child Protection Practice and Services. Munro Review of Child Protection: Final Report: A Child-Centred System.* Department of Education, London.

Department of Education (2015) *Working Together to Safeguard Children: A Guide to Inter-Agency Working to Safeguard and Promote the Welfare of Children.* Department of Education, London.

Further reading

Care Quality Commission (2009) *Safeguarding Children: A Review of Arrangements in the NHS for Safeguarding Children.* Care Quality Commission, London.

Children's Workforce Development Council (2009) The Common Assessment Framework: Early Identification, Assessment of Needs and Intervention: A Guide for Practitioners. Available at: www.cwd.council.uk

8 Family-centred care

Child outline

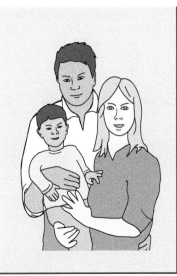

Overview of family-centred care

- UNCRC (1989) mainly Articles 3, 12, 13, 17 and 24
- It must be in the child's best interests
- Nurses need to be sufficiently skilled and experienced in order that they can adequately support, teach and empower families
- The professional acts to promote normal family functioning and autonomy
- The family is respected for the knowledge they have of their child, with the parent as the constant person in the child's life
- The diversity of family life is respected and families are not made to conform to the socially constructed norms of the institution, for example, keeping to child's routine

Key analytical skills used within nursing assessment

- Collecting information (vital signs, observation, history, parents' and child's perspective)

- Recording and reporting as a cyclical process

- Assessing and questioning information

- Considering options: deciding between different courses of action

- Planning care using problem-solving skills

- Implementing and evaluating care by interpreting and analysing information

Negotiation

- Involvement and participation by parents in the physical aspects of the child's care are voluntary and negotiated

- Involving children and young people in decision-making

- Facilitating participation through negotiation

- Having a conversation about what is required, when it needs to be done and how it will be done – before any agreement about who will do what can be made

- Writing down what is agreed, and agreeing this is subject to further negotiation

- Reviewing, evaluating, summing up

- Checking the accuracy of what has been said and agreed

Communication

- A relationship exists between the family and professional that is non-judgemental and based on honest, open communication

- Information is given and received in a way that facilitates informed decision-making for families and professionals

- There is evidence of communication, co-operation and collaboration between the family and professionals

- Parents are involved in decisions made about the child's care

- Sufficient time must be available to identify the concerns of the family

Key communication skills

Pre-admission communication for children and young people
- Written information and stories
- Information through media such as NHS, internet, television and radio

Children's nurses' key communications skills
- Observing
- Listening
- Empathizing
- Use of body language
- Use of appropriate language
- Play

Participation

- Parents must want to be involved in the care

- Nurses must be willing to share the care of the sick child with the family

- Nurses must be prepared to develop a relationship with the family and collaborate with them

- Empowering children themselves, particularly in chronic or long-term conditions

Children and Young People's Nursing Skills at a Glance, First Edition. Edited by Elizabeth Gormley-Fleming and Deborah Martin.
© 2018 John Wiley & Sons, Ltd. Published 2018 by John Wiley & Sons, Ltd.

Defining family-centred care

There is a plethora of published literature which documents the evolution of family-centred care over seven decades. The term family-centred care is synonymous with children's nursing, yet a consensus on a single definition has not been achieved.

The literature identifies that family-centred care is socially constructed and relevant to the time, culture and place in which it is practised and it has been interpreted in various models. Family-centred care considers the child or young person and their family as one unit.

Fathers also have a unique contribution to make within family-centred care. Fathers are often viewed as the breadwinner and supporting the mother. This has the potential for fathers to feel 'less important' when they may wish to participate in the care of the child.

There is a dearth of literature which considers the role of siblings within family-centred care. Siblings are likely to have the longest relationship.

Following the United Nations Convention on the Rights of the Child (UNCRC, 1989), there has been a growing acknowledgement of children and young people's rights within family-centred care.

Competence in nursing assessment

Considering the needs of the children and young people in family-centred care is enhanced by the unique and vital contributions made by their parents and carers. Without their knowledge and contributions, caring for children and young people would be more challenging.

Accurate nursing assessment underpins family-centred care and partnership working. It is a complex process which draws from a range of models, concepts and ideals. From nursing assessment it is important to identify and understand the individual child or young person, their family dynamics and the context of the family environment.

Understanding the needs of children and young people will enable children's nurses to move beyond the physical, emotional, intellectual and social assessments to facilitating participation in care.

Communication and negotiation of care

When communicating with children and young people, it is important to acknowledge the age and stage of development of the child and young person in relation to language development and vocabulary. Children's nurses should be mindful of selecting appropriate vocabulary in order that the meaning is understandable and not subjective. Children draw meaning from life experiences and do not always share their thoughts with adults. Children may interpret these terms as indicators of danger or fatality.

Research has shown that younger children prefer adults to communicate on their behalf. As children develop, they wish to communicate directly with the health professionals, however, parents may still communicate on their behalf, thus the 'child's voice' will be 'silenced' or only partially included according to parenting styles. Young people move into a position where they assume a lead in communicating with health professionals and establish an active voice.

Effective communication within family-centred care is complex and requires active listening skills. A single conversation with a family may include the child or young person and their family. Each child or young person and their family is unique and has different care needs and requires different levels of support. Therefore, it is important to negotiate the parts of care they wish to undertake. Negotiation of care should be meaningful and avoid tokenism. Negotiation requires the children's nurse to wish to share the care. Children's nurses should be mindful of the language they use. Well-meaning phrases such as 'my patient' do not indicate a readiness to share care. Children, young people and their families should not feel compelled to participate in care.

Effective communication is the basis for meaningful negotiation of care between the child or young person, the family and the children's nurse.

Participation in care

Enabling children and young people to participate in their care may be a straightforward transition. Children and young people with complex care needs can be empowered to learn new skills in order that they are less dependent on their parents for their care needs.

The literature identifies that children and young people should be active participants in their healthcare journeys. Empowering children, young people and their parents to participate in care shifts the locus of control to enable them to be active participants in their healthcare. This will be particularly important where the child has a chronic or long-term condition.

Children's nurses are in a pivotal position to teach children, young people and their families any new skill. New knowledge, information and skills will enable children and young people to become active participants in their care. In order for the child, young person and their families to learn these new skills or techniques, it is important to plan participatory experiences. The demonstration of the skills or technique should be broken down into smaller, sequential stages. The opportunity for questioning should be expected and a range of answers to anticipated questions could be prepared. As children's nurses are accountable for their actions or omission, careful consideration of the documentation of competence to undertake the skill or technique is required.

Key points
- Family-centred care should be negotiated with children, young people and their families.
- Tokenistic negotiations with children, young people and the families are inappropriate.
- The voices of children, young people and their families are vital in family-centred care.
- Participatory experiences enable children, young people and their families to be involved in new care needs.

Reference

United Nations Convention on the Rights of the Child (1989) Available at: www.unicef.org.crc

Further reading

Shields, L., Huaqiong, Z., Pratt, J., Taylor, M., Hunter. J. and Pascoe, E. (2012) Family centred care for hospitalised children aged 0–12 years. *Cochrane Database of Systematic Reviews*. DOI: 10.1002/14651858.CD004811.pub3

9 Record keeping

Main principles of the Nursing and Midwifery Council (NMC) Record-keeping Guidelines
Source: Adapted from Nursing and Midwifery Council (2015) The Code. https://www.nmc.org.uk/standards/code/

Accurate and objective → Recording of information

Protection of information → Confidentiality

Only in the child's best interest → Disclosed

Record-keeping principles

Information systems

Access to information → Privacy and permission

Ensure systems are used properly

Professional knowledge and skills → Nurses' professional duty

Record keeping as part of care planning

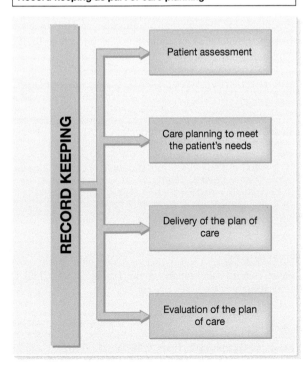

RECORD KEEPING

- Patient assessment
- Care planning to meet the patient's needs
- Delivery of the plan of care
- Evaluation of the plan of care

Using SBAR for recording handover

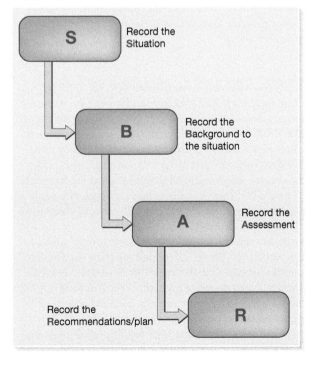

S — Record the Situation

B — Record the Background to the situation

A — Record the Assessment

R — Record the Recommendations/plan

Children and Young People's Nursing Skills at a Glance, First Edition. Edited by Elizabeth Gormley-Fleming and Deborah Martin.
© 2018 John Wiley & Sons, Ltd. Published 2018 by John Wiley & Sons, Ltd.

Record-keeping overview

Record keeping or documentation is an integral component of communication in today's healthcare climate. It is essential that good practice in record keeping is upheld and that documentation is undertaken and maintained according to local policies and recommendations from the Nursing and Midwifery Council (NMC, 2010). Keeping accurate and thorough health records is part of providing the best care for the children, young people and their families. A health record collates information about the health condition of an individual recorded by health professionals in the multi-disciplinary team (MDT).

Principles of good record keeping

The Figure provides an overview of the main areas of good record keeping taken from the NMC (2010) guidelines.

Handwriting should be legible and all entries to records should be signed, dated with a time indicated. For written records, name and job title should be printed alongside the first entry. Records should be accurate, factual and the use of abbreviations, subjective judgements and jargon avoided. It is also important to ensure that important events about a patient are recorded in a timely fashion. The term 'contemporaneous' in relation to record keeping refers to information being written at the time of the event or as soon afterwards that is possible to provide a chronological and accurate record of events. This is vitally important as it captures the reality of the events within which care was delivered and can be used in evidence in any legal proceedings.

The language used should be easily understood by those in our care and all records should be readable when photocopied or scanned. Records should not be altered or destroyed without authorization.

Details of any assessments and reviews undertaken including documentation of future planned care should be undertaken for all children and families. Where appropriate, children and their families, should be involved in the record-keeping process regarding plans and decisions.

There are certain important elements of record keeping that must be considered:

• *Confidentiality*: Nurses should be fully aware of the legal requirements and guidance regarding confidentiality, and again, ensure practice is in line with national and local policies. Discussions about those in our care should not take place where they might be overheard, and records, either paper or digital, should not be made available to others. Data protection policies must also be followed in line with this.
• *Access*: Children and families in our care have a right to ask to see their own health records and they also can ask for their information to be withheld from you or other health professionals. This should be respected unless withholding such information would cause serious harm to that person or others. Records should not be accessed to find out personal information.
• *Disclosure*: Information that can identify an individual must not be used or disclosed for purposes other than healthcare without the individual's explicit consent unless the law requires it.
• *Information systems*: Smartcards or passwords to access information systems must never be shared. Similarly, systems should not be left open to access by unauthorized persons. All systems should be used appropriately, particularly in relation to confidentiality.
• *Personal and professional knowledge and skills*: Nurses have a duty, according to the NMC (2010) 'to keep up to date with, and adhere to, relevant legislation, case law, and national and local policies relating to information and record keeping'. The ability to communicate effectively within teams is a crucial part of nursing

practice. The way information is recorded is important since other members of the MDT will rely on records at key communication points, for example, at handover, referral and in shared care.

Care plan documentation

Record keeping in the form of care plans is an important part of holistic care so that all members of the MDT are aware of the individual care needs for children and families. The Figure summarizes the four important areas for record keeping and communication between health care professionals: assessment, planning of care, delivery of nursing care and evaluation of that care. These are the components of the nursing process; this, along with planning care, is the subject of Chapter 10.

Handover documentation

Communication between nursing shifts is essential for safe and consistent care and the handover period is central to this. Clear documentation should be in place in order to hand over important information about the planned care for individual children and families. The Figure uses the SBAR mnemonic (**S**ituation-**B**ackground-**A**ssessment-**R**ecommendations) to illustrate which elements can be recorded to hand over all the essential information to the subsequent shift.

Ethico-legal issues

Nurses have a professional role and responsibility to ensure accurate record keeping in line with their code of conduct. There are also important ethico-legal issues surrounding record keeping that nurses should be aware of. Patient records are legal documents and can be used in cases of litigation against a Trust to prove the events that occurred; therefore, it is vital that all care and outcomes are clearly documented throughout the stay in hospital or the care period. At times of conflict, accurate and objective documentation is essential. Finally, where consent is obtained from patients, be this from the child or the family, it must be recorded clearly in the health records.

Key points

• Nurses have a duty to communicate effectively with their colleagues, ensuring that they have all the information they need about children and families. Record keeping, undertaken according to local and national guidelines, in an integral part of this communication process.
• Good practice in documentation is an essential process within the nursing care of children and families with ethico-legal implications.
• Accurate record keeping serves as a tool for communication in relation to the documentation of health records, for handover between shifts and the multi-disciplinary team and for care planning for children and families.

Reference

Nursing and Midwifery Council (2010) *Guidance on Professional Conduct for Nursing and Midwifery Students*. NMC, London.

Further reading

NHS Institute for Innovation and Improvement (2013) *Paediatric SBAR*. Available at: http://www.institute.nhs.uk/images//documents/SaferCare/SBAR/Pads/Paediatric_SBARv2_A5.pdf
Nursing and Midwifery Council (2015) *The Code*. Available at: https://www.nmc.org.uk/standards/code/
Royal College of Nursing (2013) *Delegating Record-keeping and Countersigning Records Guidance for Nursing Staff*. RCN, London.

10 Planning care

The nursing process

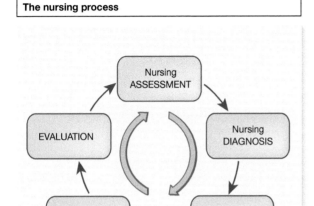

Activities of living Source: Roper et al., 2000. Reproduced with permission of Elsevier

- Maintaining a safe environment
- Communicating
- Breathing
- Eating and drinking
- Eliminating
- Personal cleansing and dressing
- Controlling body temperature
- Mobilizing
- Working and playing
- Expressing sexuality
- Sleeping
- Dying

Family-centred care model (Casey, 1988)

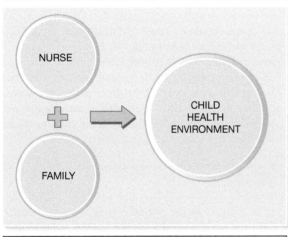

Family-centred care plan example

Problem	Goal	Intervention	Family intervention	Evaluation

Orem's self-care requisites

- ☐ The maintenance of a sufficient intake of air
- ☐ The maintenance of a sufficient intake of water
- ☐ The maintenance of a sufficient intake of food
- ☐ Satisfactory elimination functions
- ☐ The maintenance of a balance between activity and rest
- ☐ The maintenance of a balance between solitude and social integration
- ☐ The prevention of hazards of life
- ☐ The promotion of functioning and development within social groups and the desire to be normal (normacy)

Orem's (1991) self-care deficit model

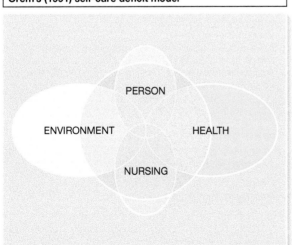

Children and Young People's Nursing Skills at a Glance, First Edition. Edited by Elizabeth Gormley-Fleming and Deborah Martin.
© 2018 John Wiley & Sons, Ltd. Published 2018 by John Wiley & Sons, Ltd.

Planning care overview

Care planning is an essential part of health care and an integral part of a nurse's role in aiming to provide continuity for the patient. There is an expectation that children and their families can trust the nurse to treat them as partners, work with them to make a holistic and systematic assessment of their needs and develop a personalized plan.

Everyone involved should be made aware of what needs to be done for any given child and family. Having individualized care plans that incorporate all aspects ensures that holistic care is given and assists the child and family to know what to expect in their care. Without a specific document delineating the plan of care, important issues are likely to be neglected. Care planning therefore provides a guide that maps out interventions. To be effective and comprehensive, the care planning process must involve all disciplines that are involved in the care of a child and family.

The nursing process

Care planning can be considered as a process and this fits well with the well-cited 'nursing process'. The nursing process is cited as a framework for problem solving but, more importantly, it assists the structured and logical planning of care on an individual basis. Initially, there were four distinct phases – assessment (and identifying problems), planning (setting goals), implementation of care, and evaluation of that care. The Figure outlines the nursing process as *five* phases with the optional addition of nursing diagnosis after assessment.

- *Assessment*: this involves gaining information about and from the child and family in order to identify their problems that require attention and intervention. The various forms of assessment have been covered in the preceding chapters in Part 1. Assessment not only identifies problems but also leads to a nursing *diagnosis*, i.e. a clinical judgement about the individual. Potential problems should also be identified and considered in light of the findings from the initial assessment.
- *Planning*: Intended outcomes and goals are set which should be realistic and achievable. These can be short-term (for example, hospital-based, emergency department) or long-term (for example, in chronic illness within the community setting). The question to ask here is, 'What needs to be done for this child?'
- *Implementation*: this is the action required or the delivery of care interventions planned, including those from others members of the multi-disciplinary team.
- *Evaluation*: The final, key phase, as this is where the nurse ensures that the care given has been effective, and checks if the goals have been achieved. If they have not, then reassessment is necessary in order to reach a positive outcome. This is why the nursing process is cyclical. Evaluation of all initial goals and plans should take place within an appropriate time frame.

Models of nursing

There are many models of nursing that can be used in conjunction with the nursing process. Used together, they are fundamental tools that serve as a framework to consider and plan the care of individual children and families. A model directs the thinking of those caring for the child in relation to the context of the health care situation. They also help direct nursing interventions and how these are given and evaluated. Three models are outlined below:

- Roper et al.'s (2000) Activities of Living Model: The Roper-Logan-Tierney Model for Nursing is a theory of nursing care based on activities of living (AoLs). The theory is used as an assessment throughout the patient's care. The theory attempts to define what living means in relation to activities of living through complete assessment leading to interventions. The AoLs should not be used as a checklist of boxes. Instead, they should be viewed as an approach to the assessment and organization of the care of the patient. A child's and a family's problems can be identified and considered within each AoL as appropriate to the individual case.
- Casey's (1988) Family-Centred Care Model: Casey's Model of Nursing focuses on the nurse working in partnership with the child and his or her family. This was one of the earliest attempts to develop a nursing model designed specifically for child health nursing. The five aspects of this nursing theory are: the child, the family, health, the environment, and the nurse. Any problem identified for an individual case should include a partnership between the nurse and family, with involvement along with interaction with the child, their health and environmental needs during illness. The Figure shows how a written care plan can incorporate family intervention.
- Orem's (1991) Self-Care Deficit Model: Similar to Casey's model, the four elements of Orem's nursing theory are the person (child/family), health, the environment, and the nurse. The theory of self-care refers to the practice of activities or requisites that an individual initiates and performs on his or her own behalf to maintain life, health, and well-being. Universal self-care requisites are associated with life processes, as well as the maintenance of the integrity of human structure and functioning. Self-care deficits exist, however, when a person becomes ill or unable to perform these requisites and maintain optimum health. Therefore, a child's problems are identified according to these requisites and whether they have any deficit under each one.

Finally, it must be emphasized how important accurate and ongoing documentation is in relation to care planning. Record keeping was covered in Chapter 9; an individual's plan of care is an integral part of this. The Nursing and Midwifery Council emphasizes that nurses should ensure healthcare records for patients or clients are accurate accounts of treatment, care planning and delivery.

Key points
- The nursing process and models of nursing care are frameworks for planning the care given to individual children and their families.
- Used in conjunction with the nursing process, a model of care directs the thinking in relation to how the child and family is viewed and so care can be planned and tailored accordingly.
- Having comprehensive and accurately documented care plans for individual patients serves as a key communication tool for all disciplines involved in the care of children and families.

References
Casey, A. A. (1988) Partnership with child and family. *Senior Nurse*, **8**(4), 8–9.
Orem, D. E. (1991) *Nursing Concepts of Practice*. Mosby, St Louis, MO.
Roper, N., Logan, W. and Tierney, A. (2000) *The Roper-Logan-Tierney Model of Nursing Based on Activities of Living*. Churchill Livingstone, London.

Further reading
Murphy, F., Williams, A. and Pridmore, J. A. (2010) Nursing models and contemporary nursing 1: their development, uses and limitations. *Nursing Times*, **106**(3), 18–20.

11 Airway and breathing

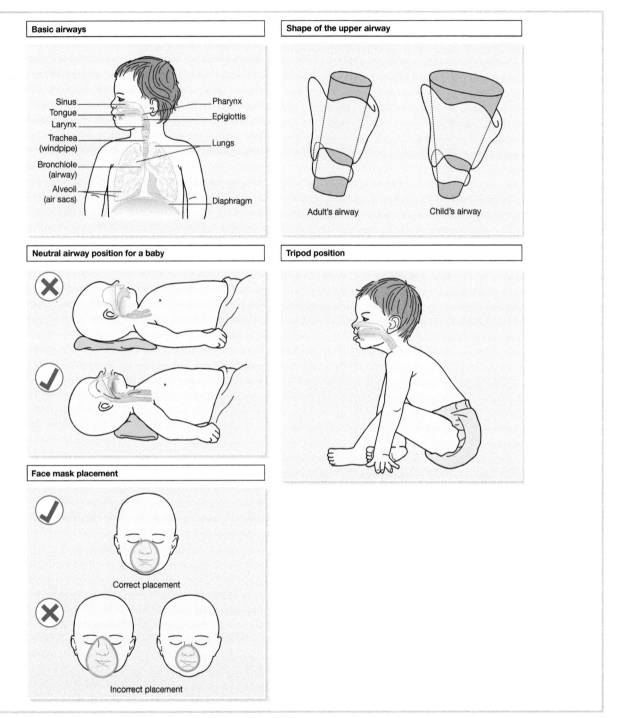

Basic airways

Sinus
Tongue
Larynx
Trachea (windpipe)
Bronchiole (airway)
Alveoli (air sacs)

Pharynx
Epiglottis
Lungs
Diaphragm

Shape of the upper airway

Adult's airway

Child's airway

Neutral airway position for a baby

Tripod position

Face mask placement

Correct placement

Incorrect placement

Airway and breathing overview

Airway is the first assessment in the systematic ABCDE approach to patient assessment: **A** = airway (c spine), **B** = breathing, **C** = circulation, **D** = disability, **E** = exposure. All aspects of the systematic approach require continuous review. The primary objective of airway assessment is to confirm an open and patent airway. Red flags are signs that warrant immediate medical review.

The basic anatomical structures which make up the upper airway are: the nose, the pharynx, the epiglottis, the larynx, the cricoid and the trachea.

Children and Young People's Nursing Skills at a Glance, First Edition. Edited by Elizabeth Gormley-Fleming and Deborah Martin.
© 2018 John Wiley & Sons, Ltd. Published 2018 by John Wiley & Sons, Ltd.

Children will predominantly present in respiratory arrest as a primary event unless there is an underlying medical condition. This respiratory response is due to the compensatory processes of children's bodies through cell oxygenation and the development of major organs, such as the heart (left ventricle) and the kidneys.

Airway needs to be simultaneously assessed with the general discriminator AVPU – Alert, Verbal, Pain, Unresponsive. This may involve waking up a sleeping child. A lowered conscious state automatically places a child's airway at risk. Understanding how the anatomy of a child's airway changes from birth to 11 years will provide the rationale for your practice. It will help to identify red flags and other key presentations that place a child at risk. The common causes of upper airway obstruction in the under-4 age group are viral illness such as croup and ingestion of foreign bodies. Additional presentations include smoke and chemical inhalation.

Difference between the child and adult airways

From birth to 6 months, babies are obligate nasal breathers which means they breathe through the nose. This is thought to be due to several structural features which are developing in this age group. The first are skeletal structures, which are a short neck and large occiput (back of head). The second are internal structures of the airway. A baby's tongue is proportionally larger than the internal surface area of their mouth. Together with a smaller pharynx, this places their tongue closer to the palate and oral airway, essentially blocking the oral airway, causing the baby to breathe through the nose. Putting all of these structures together for nursing practice, correctly positioning a baby's airway and head in a neutral position for airway is paramount. A large occiput naturally flexes the baby's head forward, causing airway occlusion. Hyper-extension will also cause occlusion. The correct placement of oxygen masks is equally fundamental to prevent compression of the external nares (nostrils).

Continuing down the airway of a small child, the epiglottis is larger and floppier than that of an adult. The larynx is higher up and more anterior and superior in position (at the front of the throat extending towards the base). This makes the airway funnel-shaped with the narrowest point at the cricoid. The trachea (windpipe) is less rigid in structure and more compliant. The adult airway in comparison is straight with better integrity. In plain terms, the airway of a small child is more at risk of collapse and obstruction than that of an adult.

Signs of airway obstruction

Understanding the development of children's airway will help to you to differentiate between a normal physiological function such as drooling in the under-6 months and drooling as sign of potential airway obstruction.

As referenced, babies under 6 months old are obligate nasal breathers therefore mouth breathing in this age group signifies moderate to severe distress. Mouth breathing accompanied by drooling is a red flag for any aged child as it indicates partial airway occlusion. Drooling means that the child is unable to swallow their secretions. Supporting your practice for airway assessment are other algorithms such as the Westerly score used in the assessment of croup. It helps to determine the severity of croup and provides guidelines for treatment.

Breathing in the lower airway

Children under the age of 8 years are termed diaphragmatic breathers due to using the diaphragm muscle to alter the thoracic pressure for ventilation. Up to this stage of development the rib cage in a small child is highly compliant and horizontal in structure, which means that thoracic movement does effectively change lung pressure.

Your assessment must include establishing respiratory effort and air entry. While the respiration rate is an important observation to monitor, the most definitive clinical indicator for a child's respiratory status is work of breathing. Is the child shallow breathing or splinting?

A child who is alert with a patent airway and normal respiratory effort will essentially have quiet breathing. It is important to know that complete airway occlusion will also present as quiet breathing, again reiterating the need to assess a child's conscious status.

Normal effort in the under-6-month age group is nasal breathing with soft abdominal effort. Nasal flaring is therefore an alert. This is the physiological response by the body to attempt to increase positive pressure and ventilation through the nares. Placing the baby's head in a neutral position will expose the suprasternal notch to allow assessment for a tracheal tug.

A simple method to examine the chest in a child of any age is to ask the parent or carer to expose their trunk. Obviously this will involve respecting the privacy and dignity of the patient. Full observation of the chest and abdomen can be made. Red flags for a child of any age are sternal recession and see-saw effort (opposite chest to abdominal rise). Placing the child in a side profile can also help to visualize the rib margins better to assess intercostal recession – drawing in air, which in isolation is termed mild-to-moderate effort.

Physical examination and physical presentations

Completing this section is physical examination. Auscultation with a stethoscope is recommended for full assessment of the upper and lower airway. But this is recognized as an advanced competence. Your assessment may include hearing an audible wheeze (heard on expiration) or stridor (heard on inspiration).

For verbal children, an easy technique is to ask them to speak a full sentence. Speech is formed through the larynx and vocal cords on expiration. A child who struggles to speak one to three words is showing airway compromise.

To conclude, the red flag or severe respiratory effort in the under-6-month age group is head bobbing – the physiological attempt to increase positive pressure using the clavicular muscles. With gross motor development, this form of respiratory distress in self-supporting children presents as the tripod position.

Key points

• Prompt treatment is required if airway obstruction is suspected.
• Simple manoeuvres, such as a head tilt or a chin lift, may be sufficient to clear the airway.
• Continued assessment is required if an airway is partially obstructed as this situation could rapidly change to a completely occluded airway.

Further reading

Department of Health (n.d.) *Spotting the Sick Child*. Available at: https://www.spottingthesickchild.com
Resuscitation Council (UK) (2011) *Paediatric Immediate Life Support*, 2nd edition. Available at: https://www.resus.org.uk

12 Circulatory assessment

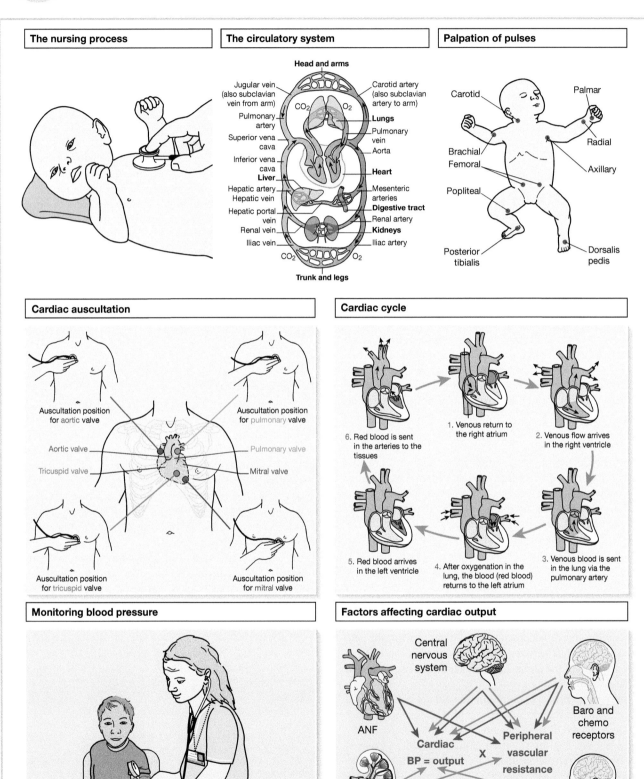

The nursing process

The circulatory system

Head and arms

Jugular vein (also subclavian vein from arm)
Carotid artery (also subclavian artery to arm)
Pulmonary artery
Lungs
CO_2 O_2
Superior vena cava
Pulmonary vein
Aorta
Inferior vena cava
Liver
Heart
Hepatic artery
Hepatic vein
Mesenteric arteries
Hepatic portal vein
Digestive tract
Renal vein
Renal artery
Kidneys
Iliac vein
Iliac artery
CO_2 O_2

Trunk and legs

Palpation of pulses

Carotid
Palmar
Radial
Brachial
Femoral
Axillary
Popliteal
Posterior tibialis
Dorsalis pedis

Cardiac auscultation

Auscultation position for aortic valve
Auscultation position for pulmonary valve
Aortic valve
Pulmonary valve
Tricuspid valve
Mitral valve
Auscultation position for tricuspid valve
Auscultation position for mitral valve

Cardiac cycle

6. Red blood is sent in the arteries to the tissues
1. Venous return to the right atrium
2. Venous flow arrives in the right ventricle
5. Red blood arrives in the left ventricle
4. After oxygenation in the lung, the blood (red blood) returns to the left atrium
3. Venous blood is sent in the lung via the pulmonary artery

Monitoring blood pressure

Factors affecting cardiac output

Central nervous system
ANF
Baro and chemo receptors
Cardiac
BP = output X Peripheral vascular resistance
Renin-angiotensin
Anti-diuretic hormone

Children and Young People's Nursing Skills at a Glance, First Edition. Edited by Elizabeth Gormley-Fleming and Deborah Martin.
© 2018 John Wiley & Sons, Ltd. Published 2018 by John Wiley & Sons, Ltd.

Circulatory assessment overview

Circulatory assessment forms part of a complete assessment of the patient and many other aspects of the infant's or child's condition will dictate parts of the cardiovascular assessment. Therefore, no information should be viewed in isolation. Given that abnormalities in fluid status can lead to deterioration, having a good understanding of the circulatory status of a patient is very important, also understanding why these changes may be significant. It is important to attempt an assessment when the child or infant is as calm as possible. Plan your approach in advance, as agitation and anxiety can lead to abnormal findings. If possible, attempt the assessment with the child sitting on the parent's or carer's lap or as close to them as possible to minimize stress in the child or infant. Much of the assessment can be gained by calmly observing the infant without a full examination, for example, consider the facial features (dysmorphic features?), also the rate and work of breathing. Use distraction, simple efforts to keep a child or infant calm will help in assessing them more accurately. Calculating cardiac output does not form part of a *basic* assessment but having an understanding of how the amount of blood each minute affects the body, via an assessment, gives a good understanding of the patient's cardiovascular function.

Cardiac output

The heart's action as a pump is to create 'cardiac output' or the amount of blood (stroke volume) pumped out of the heart in one minute. This is assessed via a cardiovascular assessment, considering perfusion, heart rate, blood pressure, pulse volume and the patient's temperature. The relevance, even to a basic assessment, is that all cellular function is primarily reliant on oxygen, which is carried via blood pumped by the heart, therefore if the heart is not pumping as well as it should, perfusion will be diminished and organ function will deteriorate accordingly. This manifests in a number of ways, three examples to be aware of are: (1) reduced urine output, indicating global dehydration or reduced renal perfusion; (2) increased (in particular) respiratory rate or effort may indicate fluid retention within the lungs, indicating cardiac failure, or may be due to a respiratory cause or due to anxiety; and (3) agitation may be because the patient is scared or due to reduced cerebral perfusion. Be mindful of the whole fluid status of the patient when making an assessment.

Factors that determine cardiac output include the cardiac function (how well the heart is working), the heart rate (HR) (the heart rate is useful for cardiac function up to a point – if a patient becomes too tachycardic, this function will fail), the amount of blood entering the ventricle (pre-load) and the amount leaving the ventricle (afterload). This is calculated using the formula:

Cardiac output stroke volume (litres/beat) × heart rate

Inspection

Using good timing, i.e. not when the patient is hungry or has just undergone a procedure, use patience and distraction if possible, take time to assess the whole child. Consider their general appearance: do they appear in good health? Are there any obvious dysmorphic features? Are there any scars or signs of previous surgery? Is there cyanosis or low SaO_2? Are they mottled? Are they sweaty? Do they appear to using an increased effort to breathe? Also how do they interact with their parent or carer? It is always important to bear in mind other parts of a child's or infant's life, for example, their social situation. Be mindful this quiet inspection may also present safeguarding concerns.

Palpation

After seeking permission to physically examine the patient, palpate pulses in the following areas: first, check radial, brachial and femoral, then attempt palmer, axillary, carotid (older children), popliteal, posterior tibialis and dorsalis pedis. This is also useful when considering sites for taking blood pressure measurements. Are pulses present? Are they even? Consider the rate, rhythm, volume and any other notable findings, for example, thrill. The apex beat is usually found in the 4th to 5th intercostal space in the mid-clavicular line. If it is not found in this position, this may be significant and requires reporting, as it may indicate a cardiac abnormality. Is the heart rate within normal limits? Attempt to palpate the liver, just below the diaphragm, usually on the right in the mid-clavicular line – this should not be palpable, a palpable liver may indicate fluid overload and needs reporting.

Auscultation

Using a stethoscope, warm the diaphragm of the bell (round disk) and auscultate the four main areas: aortic, pulmonary, tricuspid and mitral/apex, listening for heart sounds, added sounds and murmurs. Added sounds and murmurs are difficult, however, to discern, so concentrate primarily on heart sounds. First sound (S1): closing of the mitral and tricuspid valves. Second sound (S2): closure of the aortic and pulmonary valves.

Fluid balance

This should be calculated at a minimum hourly in the sicker patient, less frequently in the more stable patient. The importance of this inspection, indicating cardiac, respiratory and renal function should not be underestimated. Ensure the fluid total is taken into account in this assessment as any significant discrepancies may account for abnormalities found and will indicate a possible solution. If this is part of an initial assessment, take time to discuss the number of wet nappies an infant has had in the past 24 hours, most parents or carers will know this and it is a strong indicator regarding fluid status. At this time consider the condition of the skin and mucous membranes; decreased skin turgor is indicated when skin is gently pulled upwards and it remains in place for a few seconds – this is a significant sign of dehydration as are dry mucous membranes (mouth, eyelids), also an absence of tears in a child who appears distressed may indicate significant dehydration.

Key points

- Timing is important so a quiet, happy child is easier to examine than a hungry, upset one.
- Normal age-related values of heart rate, blood pressure and pulse volume must be known.
- Simple actions such as warm hands and a warm stethoscope will enable a more pleasant experience for the child.
- Listening to and learning heart sounds require practice and a quiet environment.

13 Measuring blood pressure

Korotkoff's sound

Korotkoff's sound	Discription
Phase 1	A clear tapping sound
Phase 2	A blowing or swishing sound
Phase 3	A softer tapping sound than phase 1
Phase 4	Sound becomes faint or muffled
Phase 5	Disappearance of all sound

Oscillometric device

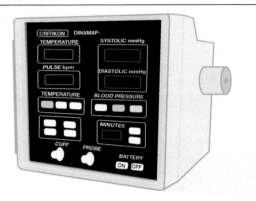

Manual sphygmomanometer

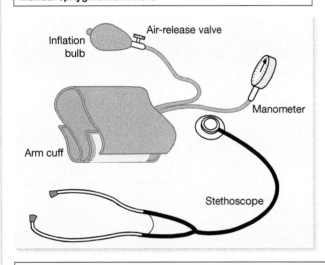

Correct position of cuff

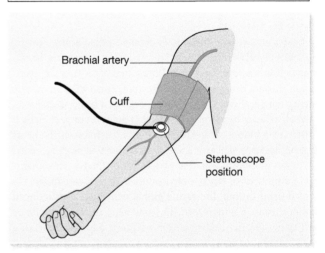

Normal blood pressure values

Discription	Normal systolic blood pressure (mmHg)	Lower limit
0 – 1 month	>60	50 – 60
1 – 12 months	80	70
1 – 10 years	90 + (2 x age in years)	70 + (2 x age in years)
>10 years	120	90

Children and Young People's Nursing Skills at a Glance, First Edition. Edited by Elizabeth Gormley-Fleming and Deborah Martin.
© 2018 John Wiley & Sons, Ltd. Published 2018 by John Wiley & Sons, Ltd.

Measuring blood pressure overview

Blood pressure may be defined as cardiac output x systemic vascular resistance. It is the pressure of the blood exerted against the walls of the arteries as the blood flows through the artery. Blood pressure should always be assessed as part of the initial assessment of an infant or child and then as the child's condition dictates. It may give an indication of cardiac function in the presence of known cardiac disease and renal function in the presence of chronic renal insufficiency. Blood pressure is recorded as systolic (contraction of left ventricle and ejection of blood into arterial vessels) over diastolic (recoil of the artery and relaxation of the heart).

It is important to note that children have the ability to compensate in the presence of a decreased cardiac output so hypotension is a late and pre-terminal sign of decompensating shock. It will require immediate treatment and the instigation of life support for the child.

Blood pressure is recorded and monitored in two ways:

* non-invasive
* invasive.

Non-invasive blood pressure measurement is performed either manually with a sphygmomanometer or an automated device. Manual recording is the gold standard in non-invasive measurement of blood pressure. However, it can be challenging to record the blood pressure of a young child with a sphygmomanometer due to their lack of cooperation and the difficulties in auscultating a brachial pulse in their cubital fossa.

Cuff size

The most important aspect in recording an infant's or a child's blood pressure is choosing the correct cuff size, whether their blood pressure (BP) is being recorded manually or electronically. The cuff size should not be determined by the manufacturer's sizing on the cuff but by the child's arm dimensions. 'undercuffing' – too narrow or too short a bladder, can lead to overestimation of BP, and 'overcuffing' – too wide or too long may lead to underestimation. The cuff should be two-thirds of the distance from the elbow to the shoulder or the upper thigh, and the bladder of the cuff should cover 100% of the circumference of the arm (Figure). The cuff size used should be documented so continuity of care can be provided.

Procedure for manual BP measurement with sphygmomanometer

* Explain the procedure to the child and family, telling them how it will feel.
* Wash your hands.
* Ensure the infant/child is resting/sitting quietly for as long possible. Ideally this should be between 1–3 minutes. The child might wish to sit on their parent's lap. BP should be recorded before any other anxiety-inducing procedures. Use diversion techniques.
* Remove restrictive clothing on arm/leg.
* Select correct size cuff.
* Ensure arm is supported and positioned at heart level.
* Apply cuff snugly around arm, ensuring that the centre of the bladder covers the brachial artery.
* Place sphygmomanometer at eye level.
* Palpate for brachial pulse.
* Close air escape valve and inflate cuff until radial pulse can no longer be palpated. Continue to inflate cuff to another 20 mmHg higher than estimated systolic pressure.
* Place diaphragm of stethoscope gently over pulse point of brachial artery, ensuring it is not tucked under edge of cuff.
* Release air valve slowly to deflate the cuff-2–3 mmHg per second.
* Note the first Korotkoff's sound – a clear tapping sound, and record as systolic value. Record the diastolic pressure as the fourth Korotkoff sound – a low-pitched, muffled sound for children up to 12 years of age. Record the fifth Korotkoff's sound – the disappearance of all sound for children aged 13–18 years.
* Remove cuff and replace child's clothing.
* Document readings on observation chart and in care records, noting limb, position, cuff size and method of measurement.
* Wash hands and clean equipment and store correctly.

Procedure for manual BP measurement with oscillometry

* You must be familiar with the operating instructions of the device available. This device must be validated.
* Apply the correctly sized cuff to the child's upper limb.
* Inflate as per instructions. It is important to keep the child as still as possible as the machine will pump to a pre-determined level initially, so if the child is upset and moving their limb, most automated devices tend to pump to a higher pressure on subsequent inflation attempts which may distress the child even more.
* Allow the cuff to deflate, note the digital reading on the display.

Invasive procedure

Invasive recording involves the insertion of an arterial line into the child which is then connected to a monitoring system. This is only practised in critical care area normally.

Key points
* Cuff size is essential in maintaining accurate readings.
* A single measurement of blood pressure is never sufficient for initiating treatment.
* Factors impacting on the measurement of blood pressure, such as medication taken, pain, or behaviour must be considered and noted.

Further reading

http://www.bhsoc.org/resources/children-young-people/

14 Assessment of pain

Physiological changes in children and infants due to pain

Vital sign	Child	Neonate and infant
Heart rate	Tachycardia	Tachycardia but may also have bradycardia
Respiratory rate	Tachypnoea	Tachypnoea but may lead to apnoea
Blood pressure	Hypertension	Hypertension
Blood glucose	Elevated	Elevated
Skin colour	Pallor	Pallor, palmar sweating

Self-reported pain assessment tool: faces pain rating scale

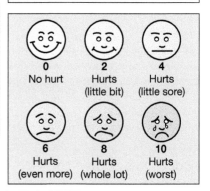

Self-reported pain assessment tools: visual analogue and ladder scales

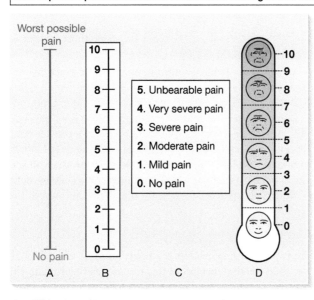

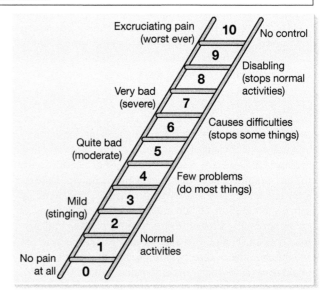

Behavioural pain assessment in an infant

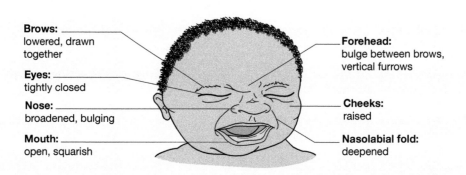

Brows: lowered, drawn together

Eyes: tightly closed

Nose: broadened, bulging

Mouth: open, squarish

Forehead: bulge between brows, vertical furrows

Cheeks: raised

Nasolabial fold: deepened

Pain assessment overview

Pain assessment is essential to enable effective pain management. It also provides the foundations for further care. Pain management in infants and children is complex. This is due to factors such as their level of cognition, their ability to communicate, prior experience, fear and severity of their illness. Children with cognitive impairment, neonates and infants require additional consideration of assessment of their pain.

Assessing pain

There are numerous pain assessment tools available to assist with the accurate assessment of the child's pain level. Self-reporting is the gold standard, however, not all children are able to communicate verbally. Physiological signs and behaviour must be considered for those children who are unable to articulate their pain. Pain assessment must be holistic and involve the parents/carers.

A systematic approach using the QUESTT model should be used:

Q = question the child about their pain and how they are feeling.
U = use an age-appropriate pain assessment tool.
E = evaluate their behaviour and physiological signs.
S = secure the involvement of parents/carers.
T = take the cause of the pain into account, what procedures has the child had?
T = take action: give treatment and evaluate.

Pain assessment tools

The correct tool must be identified and used if pain is to be assessed accurately. Pain assessment tools are either behavioural tools or self-report tools. The tool should be appropriate to the age, development and level of understanding of the child. Children who are cognitively impaired and neonates/infants will require a tool that measures physiological indicators as well as their behaviour.

Behavioural assessment

Behaviour is a very useful measure of pain in children who are pre- or non-verbal. To assess a child's behaviour, the nurse will need to stand close to the child and observe their behaviour in accordance with the cues on the assessment tool. Some of these behaviours may be reported by parents/carers. The behaviours that child may exhibit are:

- restlessness
- guarding the area affected
- unusual posture
- crying, screaming
- pulling at the affected area
- more clingy than usual
- head banging
- biting fingers
- irritability
- not feeding, decreased appetite
- anorexia
- stiffness and reluctance to move
- pulling away
- lack of interest in toys
- lethargy
- interrupted sleep pattern
- rocking

- arching back
- clenching hands
- toe flexion.

Examples of behavioural pain assessment tools are:

- FLACC
- CRIES
- the Paediatric Pain Profile (PPP)
- the Liverpool Infant Distress Scale (LIDS)

FLACC

F = facial expression
L = leg movement
A = activity
C = cry
C = consolability

CRIES

C = cries
R = requires increased oxygen saturation
I = increased vital signs
E = expression
S = sleepiness

Paediatric Pain Profile (PPP)

This behavioural tool is a 20-item behaviour rating scale and was designed for children with cognitive impairment. It involves the parents as equal carers, and they are required to complete the initial assessment of their child. It recognizes the expertise of parents in assessing their child's pain.

Liverpool Infant Distress Scale (LIDS)

This tool is for use following neonatal or infant surgery. It requires observations of the following: facial expression, sleep pattern, cry quality and cry quantity, spontaneous movement and excitability, flexion of fingers and toes, and tone.

Physiological assessment

Physiological assessment involves both measuring vital signs and also noting the child's appearance. Heart rate, blood pressure, respiratory rate, blood glucose and oxygen saturations should be measured and documented. The child's colour should be noted and their skin touched to feel for sweat. Physiological indicators of pain are identified in the table in the Figure.

Self-reported assessment

Self-reporting is the gold standard. This should be the preferred choice for children aged 4 years and upwards. The best-known self-reported pain assessment tools are visual analogue or number scales. Explanation of the relevant assessment tool is required if the assessment is to be accurate.

Key points
- Pain behaviours may not always be obvious so subtle signs should be noted.
- Children may try to hide their level of pain due to fear of further interventions.
- Assessment is an ongoing requirement of effective pain management.
- A sleeping child may be in pain.

15 Moving and handling

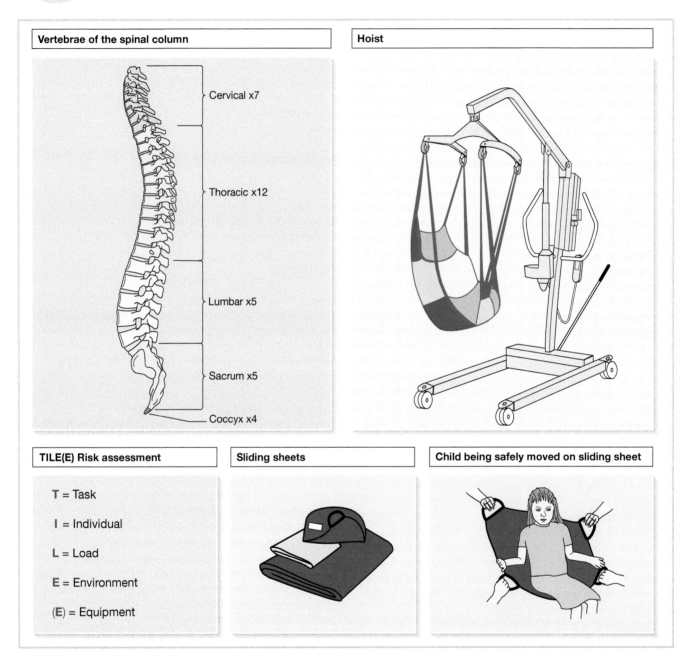

Vertebrae of the spinal column

Cervical x7

Thoracic x12

Lumbar x5

Sacrum x5

Coccyx x4

Hoist

TILE(E) Risk assessment

T = Task

I = Individual

L = Load

E = Environment

(E) = Equipment

Sliding sheets

Child being safely moved on sliding sheet

Moving and handling overview

Each day, health care professionals are moving and handling a variety of items. This can range from small pieces of equipment, moving beds and trolleys or the manual handling of infants, children and young people. Each of these activities has their own challenges and can potentially cause harm to both the health care practitioner and the patient. The aim of any moving and handling procedure is to minimize the risk to its lowest practicable level. In order to achieve this, the health care practitioner must assess, discuss, plan, and evaluate each activity to be undertaken. Each practitioner must be knowledgeable in the current legislation for manual handling practices and policies as well as have

a basic understanding of the musculoskeletal injury associated with the particular tasks that will be carried out.

Legislation

There is a considerable amount of legislation that pertains to moving and handling in the workplace. In summary, employers have general health and safety responsibilities where they are required to avoid the need for hazardous manual handling, must assess the risk of injury from any hazardous manual handling and reduce the risk of injury where it is reasonably practicable.

The employee also has a duty to adhere to this legislation. Each employee should avoid manual handling duties as far as is

Children and Young People's Nursing Skills at a Glance, First Edition. Edited by Elizabeth Gormley-Fleming and Deborah Martin.
© 2018 John Wiley & Sons, Ltd. Published 2018 by John Wiley & Sons, Ltd.

reasonably possible, assess the risk associated with each manual handling task, and must use training and equipment that have been provided for them by the employer.

Risk assessment

To work safely, it is necessary to identify what is appropriate for each child, whatever their age, at each specific time. This often entails determining what the task actually is, whether it needs to happen, how many people need to be involved, and what equipment, if any, is necessary. A risk assessment is not about creating huge amounts of paperwork, but rather about identifying sensible measures to control the risks involved in any moving and handling procedure. One form of risk assessment that is commonly used in patient handling is TILE(E).

TILE(E)

T = task: Children frequently require repetitive moving and handling from place to place, and accessing them can make the job more difficult as they are often on the floor, or at a lower level, i.e. in a cot. All these factors increase the risks associated with completing the task. Children are rarely still, their weights vary considerably and the health care practitioners are often required to lift from an awkward angle, further increasing the risk of injury.

I = individual: The individual pertains to the health care practitioner and not the child. The individual must be dressed appropriately, be aware of their own strengths and limitations, including fatigue and any pre-existing musculoskeletal injuries or conditions.

L = load: Health care practitioners must learn to recognize loads where the weight, shape and circumstances might cause potential injuries. Unfamiliar loads or patients should be treated with caution.

E = environment: Is there enough space to complete the activity? Is there adequate lighting to perform the activity safely? Consider the temperature of the space and if the floors or surfaces are slippery, uneven or carpeted.

(E) = (equipment): Equipment is there to reduce the physical effort and risk of injury. However, you should only use equipment that you have been trained to use.

Once a TILE(E) risk assessment has been completed and the activity undertaken, suitable documentation MUST be completed. Documentation of both clinical reasoning and activities undertaken is a legal requirement, it helps to enhance communication between staff, guide the safe handling of others and provide evidence and justification should your handling ever be questioned by others.

Anatomy and physiology

The spine is the central composition of the skeleton. It consists of 33 vertebrae, each pair with an intervertebral disc between them. The intervertebral disc has four main functions: (1) it acts as a shock absorber; (2) it acts as a spacer between vertebrae; (3) it reduces friction during movement; and (4) it limits excessive movement.

The most commonly injured areas of the spine are the cervical and lumbar regions due to their mobility, position and lack of protection. The disc can be damaged by mechanical changes, it can rupture suddenly (a slipped disc), which can be due to either direct trauma or more commonly a cumulative injury which occurs over time.

The correct posture in any physical activity is one which does the following:

- maintains the natural curvature of the spine;
- maintains the balance of the body;
- minimizes the level of stress on the spine.

Therefore, when manual handling, think about the following:

- Maintain a natural upright posture wherever possible, keeping your spine in line.
- Create a good stable base with your legs and feet, adopt a power position.
- Keep any load as close to your centre of gravity as possible.

Principles of safe manual handling

Here are some basic principles to adopt when considering any moving and handling manoeuvres.

- Is it possible to avoid the activity altogether?
- If it is not possible, has a risk assessment been undertaken?
- Have suitable safe systems been put in place – number of people and equipment?
- Rather than lifting, consider other movements, such as sliding, pushing, pulling or rolling.
- Think before lifting and handling.
- Keep the load close to the waist.
- Adopt a stable position.
- Get a good hold.
- Start in a good posture.
- Don't flex the back any further while lifting.
- Avoid twisting the back or leaning sideways.
- Keep the head up when handling.
- Move smoothly.
- Don't lift or handle more than can easily be managed.

Equipment

Equipment should be used to reduce the load on staff, should be easy to operate and should be in good condition through regular maintenance. Where equipment is provided for manual handling, operators must be trained in its use.

Types of equipment

Reason to move or handle	Equipment
Aids to be used to assist with sitting to standing	Raised, tip-up chairs or toilet seats, grab rails
Aids to encourage independent transfer	Transfer boards, sliding boards, turntables
Aids to be used for bed mobility	Sliding sheets; hoist, bed ladder
Aids for transfer	Sliding sheets; hoists and slings
Aids for bathing	Bath seats, bath hoists

Hoists

There are various types and makes of hoists in use for children and young people: ceiling, track, standing, bath and walking hoists. All hoists use slings and these should be specifically measured for each patient, cleaned and maintained as per the manufacturer's guidelines. When using the hoist, staff must ensure that they have had suitable training, that the hoist has been serviced and load tested as per the manufacturer's guidelines. Each child and their family should be fully briefed on why the hoist is needed and consent obtained.

Key points
- All manual handling of infants, toddlers and children has the potential to cause harm to the lifter, irrespective of their size.
- Safety is paramount when using equipment and the distress of the child should be considered before any moving is considered.

16 Measuring temperature

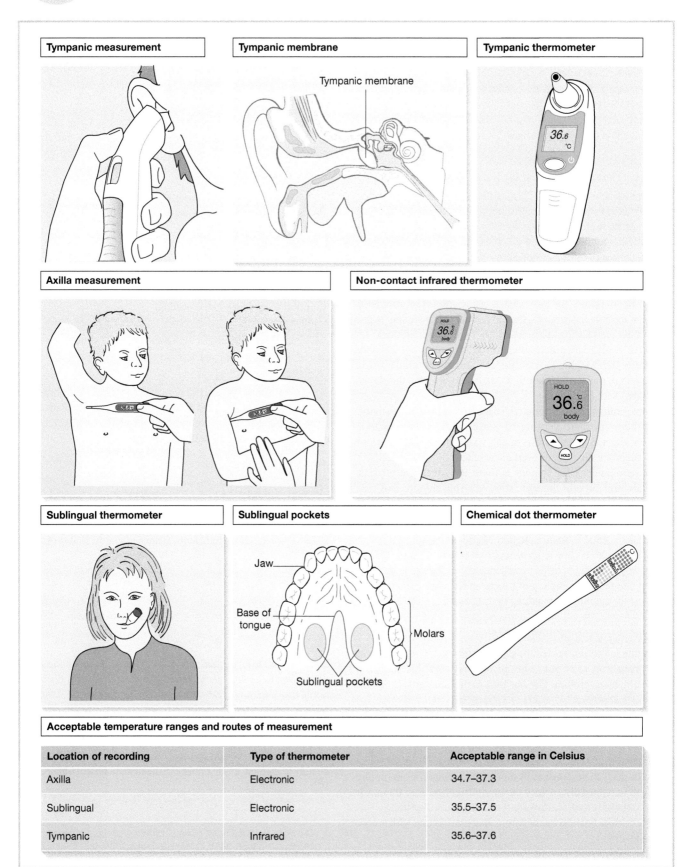

Tympanic measurement

Tympanic membrane

Tympanic membrane

Tympanic thermometer

36.6 °C

Axilla measurement

Non-contact infrared thermometer

HOLD 36.6 °C body

HOLD 36.6 °C body

Sublingual thermometer

Sublingual pockets

Jaw

Base of tongue

Molars

Sublingual pockets

Chemical dot thermometer

Acceptable temperature ranges and routes of measurement

Location of recording	Type of thermometer	Acceptable range in Celsius
Axilla	Electronic	34.7–37.3
Sublingual	Electronic	35.5–37.5
Tympanic	Infrared	35.6–37.6

Children and Young People's Nursing Skills at a Glance, First Edition. Edited by Elizabeth Gormley-Fleming and Deborah Martin.
© 2018 John Wiley & Sons, Ltd. Published 2018 by John Wiley & Sons, Ltd.

Measuring temperature overview

Fever is a common symptom in infants and young children. Measuring temperature accurately is an important clinical skill as an increase in body temperature may be indicative of illness. Body temperature is a precisely controlled homeostatic mechanism. When an increase in body temperature occurs, this is as a result of the body's natural defence mechanisms attempting to repair itself by increasing its metabolic rate and making it a hostile environment for invading pathogens.

A normal core body temperature for a newborn infant will be between 36.5°C and 37.6°C. In an older child, a temperature between 36.5°C and 37.5°C is normal. A temperature of more than 37.5°C is defined as pyrexia. Accurate assessment of body temperature is an important part of the baseline assessment of the infant and child and the ongoing measurement indicates their responsiveness to treatment.

Clinical hypothermia is a core body temperature of less than 35°C. It may be defined as mild, moderate, deep or profound. Hypothermia may be as a result of prolonged exposure to cold, drug-induced or metabolic disorders.

Hyperthermia is a significant rise in body temperature that is not attributable to infection. Some of the possible causes of hyperthermia are drug reaction, stroke, malignant hyperpyrexia or a malignancy.

Choice of procedure

The age and preference of the child will determine how the temperature will be measured. The correct thermometer and site should be used when possible. Both of these will determine the reading (see table in the Figure).

- *Infants under 4 weeks of age:* use electronic thermometer in the axilla.
  - *Infants aged 4 weeks–5 years:*
  - electronic thermometer in the axilla;
  - chemical dot thermometer in the axilla;
  - infrared tympanic thermometer.
- *5 years +:* axilla or sublingual route.

For repeated measurements of temperature it is not advised to use the chemical dot thermometers.

Equipment

thermometer
protective disposable cover
disinfectant wipes
observation chart

Make yourself familiar with the manufacturer's instructions for whichever device you are using.

Procedure

Explain the procedure to the child and their parents. Consent should be obtained at this point.

- *Axilla measurement:* loosen clothing around this area. Remove thermometer probe from base unit and place protective cover over probe. Ensure correct mode is set on base unit. Place probe in the mid-axilla and hold in place. Ensure child keeps upper arm down and in contact with their chest wall. When audible alarm sounds, ask child to lift arm up and remove probe.
- If a *chemical dot thermometer* is being used, ensure the chemical active strip is placed facing the torso and leave in situ for three minutes as per manufacturer's instructions.
- *Tympanic measurement:* Children < 1 year of age:
  - Gently pull the pinna of the ear straight back and for children > 1 year of age, pull the pinna up and back. This will enable the ear canal to be straightened so the temperature will be recorded from the tympanic membrane as it will be in direct line of sight with the probe. Cover the probe with a disposable cover and insert gently into the ear canal and press the button to begin the measurement. When the audible alarm sounds, remove the probe from the ear canal, note the reading and dispose of the probe.
  - *Sublingual:* Place the probe into the sublingual pocket under the tongue and remove when the audible alarm is heard. This route should not be used if the child has had recent food or fluids to drink or if the child is unable to hold the thermometer in the sublingual pocket.
  - Once the probe has been removed, dispose of the probe cover in the appropriate clinical waste bin, clean the device as per manufacturer's instructions and return it to its base.
  - Wash your hands.
- Document the temperature in the patient's chart, noting the site and type of thermometer used. Note trends and correlate measurement with other clinical measurements (e.g. heart rate). Report abnormalities and implement care as per care plan.

Key points

- Preparation of the child and communication are essential in order to gain the child's co-operation, thereby enabling correct measurements to be recorded.
- The general appearance and behaviour of the child should be noted during the measurement of temperature and considered if the temperature is abnormal.
- Incorrect positioning of the probe, both in the ear canal and mid-axilla, is the most common error when measuring temperature.

Further reading

National Institute for Health Care Excellence (2013) *Fever in Under 5s: Assessment and Initial Management.* Clinical Guideline CG160. London: NICE.

17 Weight, BMI, height/length and head circumference

BMI categories

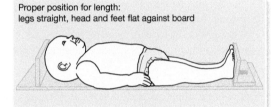

Category	BMI
Normal	19–27
Overweight	28–30
Obese	30–40
Morbidly obese	>40

Correct position for measuring length of infant

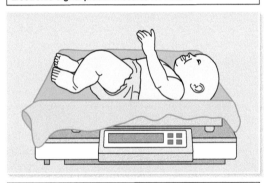

Proper position for length:
legs straight, head and feet flat against board

Electronic digital platform scales for infants

Measuring weight in an older child – standing

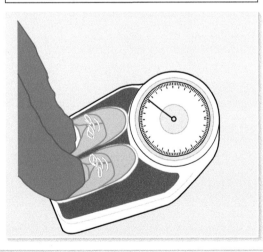

Correct position for measuring height

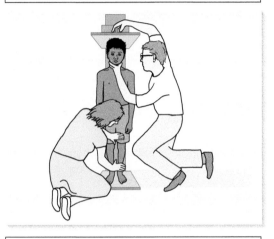

Head circumference measurement

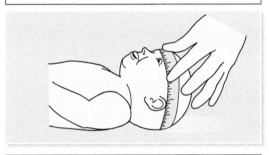

Sitting weighing scales

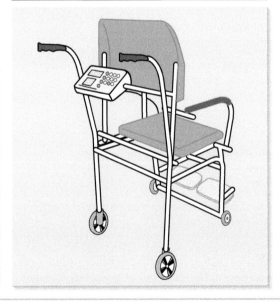

Weight, BMI, height/length and head circumference overview

Accurate measurement of height, length, weight, head and chest circumference is a vital part in the overall assessment of the infant and child in order to assure health and identify nutritional status and the impact of disease on the child. Measurements of at least two parameters are required in order to accurately assess growth. This information must then be plotted on to the relevant growth charts for the child's age and sex before it can be interpreted.

Every infant and child should have their growth assessed when accessing a health care provision.

Children and Young People's Nursing Skills at a Glance, First Edition. Edited by Elizabeth Gormley-Fleming and Deborah Martin.
© 2018 John Wiley & Sons, Ltd. Published 2018 by John Wiley & Sons, Ltd.

Weight

Weight is measured with an age-appropriate scale: an electronic digital platform scale for an infant. This should measure weight to the nearest 10 g for a child. Depending on their condition, a standing or sitting scale that will measure to the nearest 100 g should be used for an older child.

Accuracy in weighing the infant and child and the documentation of that weight are important as their medication and fluid requirement will be calculated on that weight.

The scale must be calibrated in accordance with the hospital policy and the manufacturer's instructions.

Infants should be weighed naked, toddlers in their undergarments and children in their outdoor clothing with heavy items and shoes removed. Parental involvement is key at this point to reassure the child and to keep them calm and co-operative. A warm, private area is required for undertaking this procedure.

If child is wearing a prosthetic device or other medical device that cannot be removed, this needs to be noted when documenting the weight.

Procedure for weighing infants

• Place infant on scale and remain close at hand. Place your hand lightly above their body.
• Distract the infant and note reading when the infant stops moving.
• Record the weight to the nearest 10 g.
• If repeated measurements are required, it is important to weigh at the same time every day.
• Document the weight on the percentile chart and in the care records.
• Clean scale in accordance with hospital policy and manufacturer's instructions.
• Replace paper sheet.

Procedure for weighing child

• Ask the child to stand still on weighing scale. It may be necessary to provide a distraction technique.
• Child may be weighed standing or on sitting scales.
• Note weight to nearest 100 g.
• Document the weight on the percentile chart and in the care records.

Body mass index (BMI)

The body mass index (BMI) is used in the assessment of growth in contemporary practice as the prevalence of obesity in childhood is increasing. It is considered to be an accurate determinant in quantifying obesity, and the BMI is categorized as normal, overweight, obese or morbidly obese.

Body mass index is determined by the calculation of weight in kilogrammes/height in metres^2.

$$BMI = \frac{\text{Weight in kilogrammes}}{\text{Height in metres}^2}$$

For example: a child is 20.5 kg and 94 cm in height. The height needs to be in metres^2 so when converted it is 0.8836 m^2.

$$\text{weight} = \frac{20.5}{0.8836}$$

BMI = 23.2, which is in the normal category (see table in Figure).

Height and length

In children under 2 years of age, length should be measured even after they have developed the ability to stand independently.

Length

• Remove any hats, hair decorations, footwear and nappy.
• It is helpful if the parents can distract the infant but if the infant becomes upset, it is wise to stop the procedure.
• Hold the infant's head in the midline and gently push down on the knees until straight.
• Position the heels of the feet on the footboard and record the length to the nearest millimetre.
• Repeat for accuracy.
• Plot the measurement on the appropriate percentile chart and in the care records, making sure they are dated and signed.

Height

• From the age of 2 years and if standing independently, children may have their height recorded upright with a stadiometer.
• Remove hair decorations, hat and footwear.
• Stand child straight with back to the wall and their head should be erect in the midline position.
• The child's shoulders, buttocks and heels should touch the wall and the outer cantus of the eye should be on the same horizontal plane as the external auditory canal.
• Ensure feet are flat on the floor.
• Move headpiece down to touch crown.
• Note the height reading to nearest millimetre on the indicator.
• Document height reading on the percentile chart and the care records.

Head circumference

Infants and children have their head circumference measured at birth and again at 6–8 weeks. Children up to the age of 3 years or those with questionable head size should have their head circumference recorded at regular intervals. Head circumference is a measure of the size of the skull in relation to brain size.

• A disposable, flexible, non-stretch measuring tape with centimetre and millimetre markings should be used.
• Remove any hair decorations and hats.
• Wrap tape around the head at the supraorbital prominence, above the ears and around the occipital prominence, taking care to prevent a paper cut.

• Record the circumference to the nearest 0.5 cm.
• Repeat measurement three times at slightly different points.
• Dispose of tape and wash your hands
• Plot on the percentile chart and in the care records.

Key points
• Growth is measured on at least two parameters.
• Measurements must be plotted on the correct centile chart if abnormalities are to be identified.
• Faltering growth will only be identified through regular measurements.

Further reading

Royal College of Paediatrics and Child Health, UK–WHO Growth Charts, 0–18 years. Available at: http://www.rcpch.ac.uk/growth-charts

18 Blood glucose monitoring

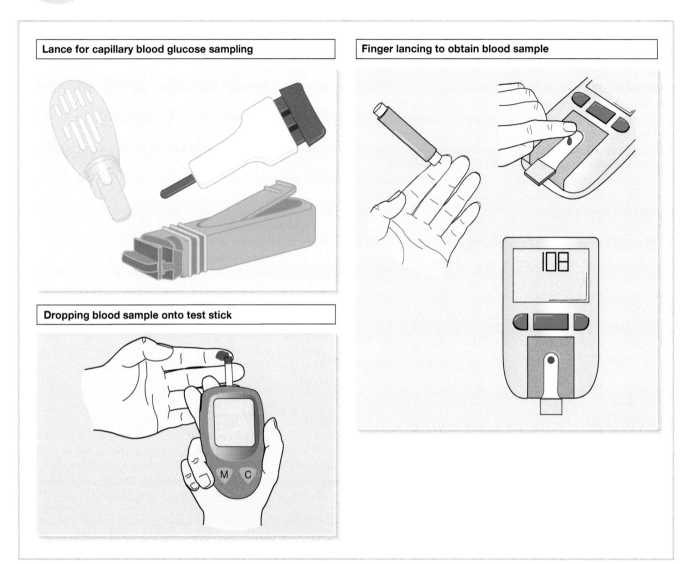

Lance for capillary blood glucose sampling

Finger lancing to obtain blood sample

Dropping blood sample onto test stick

Children and Young People's Nursing Skills at a Glance, First Edition. Edited by Elizabeth Gormley-Fleming and Deborah Martin.
© 2018 John Wiley & Sons, Ltd. Published 2018 by John Wiley & Sons, Ltd.

Blood glucose monitoring overview

What is being tested? Glucose is a simple sugar, which is the main source of energy for the body. The carbohydrates we eat are broken down into glucose, among other sugars. Glucose is absorbed by the small intestine, and then circulated through the body.

Glucose is vital for energy production; the brain and nervous system cells rely on glucose and can only function when the glucose levels in the blood remain within a certain range.

Glucose and insulin

The body cannot use glucose without the help of insulin. Insulin is a hormone produced by the pancreas and acts as a 'vehicle' to control the transport of glucose into the body's cells. After a meal, the blood glucose level rises, and insulin is excreted from the pancreas to lower it. The amount of insulin that is released is dependent upon the content of the meal.

Why would you test blood glucose levels?

This test may be used as part of a routine examination in people with increased thirst, increased urination, tiredness, blurred vision, slow healing infections, sweating, trembling, anxiety, confusion, fainting episodes, diabetes management or initial diagnosis, impaired conscious level and diarrhoea and vomiting. Blood glucose monitoring is also recommended in nil by mouth patients receiving only IV fluids for longer than 12 hours, post-operative patients, patients on medications that are known to affect blood sugar levels such as diazoxide, and patients with metabolic or endocrine conditions. Neonatal factors that might require blood glucose testing include intrauterine growth retardation, pre-term infants, infants of insulin-dependent mothers, or hypothermic babies.

How is the test performed?

A blood sample is required to complete this test. First, wash and ensure the chosen site is clean and free from glucose contamination. A drop of blood is taken from a finger/toe by using a small lancet needle. The blood is then 'absorbed' onto a glucose test strip, and a device called a glucose meter is used to measure the glucose in the blood.

In each test strip, a chemical called glucose oxidase reacts with the glucose in the blood sample and creates an acid called gluconic acid.

The glucose meter then runs an electronic current through the blood sample on the strip, and this determines how much glucose is in the sample. This number is then relayed on the screen of the device, telling you the patient's blood glucose level.

Normal blood glucose levels

The blood sugar level is the amount of glucose present in the blood. The reading obtained is expressed as millimoles per litre (mmol/l). The normal blood sugar level in people with stable blood sugars is 4–8 mmol/l.

Hyperglycaemia vs hypoglycaemia

A high blood sugar level is known as hyperglycaemia, i.e., a reading above 8 mmol/litre. There are several reasons for high blood glucose levels, including infection, stress, medication use, such as steroids, increased consumption of certain food stuffs such as cakes and biscuits, and if the patient is diabetic, then insufficient medication or problems with the injection technique or injection sites.

A low blood sugar level is known as hypoglycaemia, i.e. a reading less than 4 mmol/litre. The reasons for low blood sugar can include fasting or skipped meals, increased or unexpected exercise, alcohol intake, dehydration, and if the patient is diabetic, then too much insulin or problems with the injection technique or injection sites.

Why do blood glucose levels needs to be controlled?

Bodily functions rely on the use of glucose for energy. Sudden episodes of high or low blood sugars can be life-threatening and can cause organ failure, brain damage, coma and death.

High blood glucose levels present in the blood can damage the blood vessels. Over a sustained period of time, poorly controlled blood sugar levels can increase your chances of damaging the blood vessels. Blood glucose monitoring in diabetic patients is often performed by specialist practitioners.

Recommended reading and information on diabetes, diabetes control and management of hypoglycaemia and hyperglycaemia can be found at: www.diabetes.co.uk

Key points

- Training to emphasize the point of patient care testing of blood glucose is essential.
- The procedure should not cause distress to the child.
- Injection sites should be rotated.

19 Skin integrity

NPUAP-EPUAP classification
Source: Adapted from National Pressure Ulcer Advisory Panel, European Pressure Ulcer Advisory Panel and Pan Pacific Pressure Injury Alliance. *Prevention and treatment of Pressure Ulcers: Quick Reference Guide*. Emily Haesler (Ed.). Cambridge Media: Osborne Park, Western Australia; 2014

Category/Stage I: Non-blanchable redness of intact skin
Intact skin with non-blanchable erythema of a localized area usually over a bony prominence. Discoloration of the skin, warmth, oedema, hardness or pain may also be present. Darkly pigmented skin may not have visible blanching

Category/Stage II: Partial thickness skin loss or blister
Partial thickness loss of dermis, presenting as a shallow open ulcer with a red pink wound bed, without slough. May also present as an intact or open/ruptured serum-filled or sero-sanginous-filled blister

Category/Stage III: Full thickness skin loss (fat visible)
Full thickness tissue loss. Subcutaneous fat may be visible but bone, tendon or muscle are not exposed. Some slough may be present. May include undermining and tunnelling

Category/Stage IV: Full thickness tissue loss (muscle/bone visible)
Full thickness tissue loss with exposed bone, tendon or muscle. Slough or escher may be present. Often includes undermining and tunnelling

Classification in pictures I–IV
Source: By Nanoxyde [GFDL (http://www.gnu.org/copyleft/ftl.html) or CC BY-SA 3.0 (http://creativecommons.org/licenses/by-ses/by-sa/3.0)], via Wikimedia Commons

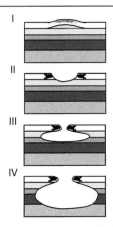

Documentation

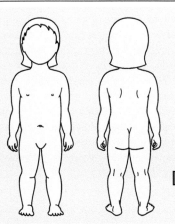

Gradings I–V skin appearance
Source: National Pressure Ulcer Advisory Panel, European Pressure Ulcer Advisory Panel and Pan Pacific Pressure Injury Alliance. *Prevention and treatment of Pressure Ulcers: Quick Reference Guide*. Emily Haesler (Ed.). Cambridge Media: Osborne Park, Australia; 2014. 3D diagrams are from the International NPUAP/EPUAP pressure ulcer classification system

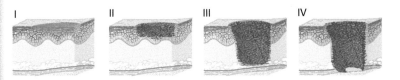

Lesion	Date observed	Description	Outcome	Date of reassessment

Paediatric Glamorgan scale
Source: Adapted from Willock et al. (2009)

Risk Factor	Score
Neonate cannot be moved or deterioration in condition/under general anaesthetic 2 hours	20
Unable to change position without assistance /cannot control body movements	15
Some mobility	10
Normal mobility for age	0
Equipment/objects/hard surfaces pressing or rubbing on skin	15
Significant anaemia	1
Persistent pyrexia	1
Poor peripheral perfusion (cold extremities/capillary refill ≥2–3 seconds/cool mottled skin	1
Inadequate nutrition	2
Low serum albumin	1
Scores: 0: No risk >10: At risk >15: High risk >20: Very high risk Plan care accordingly	

For full tool and details, see Willock et al. (2009)

The Braden Q scale for children
Source: Adapted from Noonan et al. (2011)

Intensity/duration of pressure					Score
Score-	1	2	3	4	
Mobility	Completely immobile	Very limited	Slightly limited	No limitations	
Activity	Bedbound	Chair fast	Walks occasionally	No limitations	
Sensory perception	Completely limited	Very limited	Slightly limited	No impairment	
Skin tolerance and structure					
Moisture	Constantly moist	Very moist	Occasionally moist	Rarely moist	
Friction	Significant problem	Problem	Potential problem	No apparent problem	
Nutrition	Very poor	Inadequate	Adequate	Excellent	
Tissue perfusion and oxygenation	Extremely compromised	Compromised	Adequate	Excellent	
				TOTAL=	

For full scale and details, see Noonan et al. (2011)

Children and Young People's Nursing Skills at a Glance, First Edition. Edited by Elizabeth Gormley-Fleming and Deborah Martin.
© 2018 John Wiley & Sons, Ltd. Published 2018 by John Wiley & Sons, Ltd.

Skin integrity overview

The prevention and treatment of pressure ulcers and maintenance of skin integrity in children are fundamental nursing care skills. Pressure ulcers are often considered a problem in the adult population; however, pressure ulcers also occur in the paediatric field. Prevention and management of pressure ulcers and best practice in skin care are multifaceted. One must understand the underlying physiology of skin and skin damage, the factors responsible for skin damage or ulcer development, and the factors that put infants and children at risk of poor skin integrity. Accurate assessment, documentation, prevention, and treatment are all important factors in the maintenance of skin integrity.

Risk factors that have been identified include: immobility, neurological impairment, impaired perfusion, decreased oxygenation, poor nutritional status, presence of infection and excess moisture. Even in the best of circumstances, and with preventative measures in place, skin breakdown can still occur.

Pressure ulcers are localized areas of tissue destruction occurring from soft tissue being compressed by external surfaces and bony prominences. This starves the skin of oxygen and essential nutrition. Pressure ulcers have different stages, according to the National Pressure Ulcer Advisory Panel (NPUAP). Being familiar with these stages is a sound starting point for nurses to understand what they see and then to intervene appropriately. Accurate assessment and documentation are essential parts of determining the course of treatment. The Figure outlines the key areas to document, should any skin breakdown at whatever stage occur. Skin care and assessment should also be part of a child's care plan, which includes regular reassessment and evaluation at appropriate time intervals.

However, a fundamental principle to remember is that early assessment of the risk factors associated with the development of pressure ulcers is essential in their prevention. The most common sites for pressure ulcer development in children include the buttocks, sacrum, ears, heels, elbows, malleolus and lumbar spine. In the neonatal population, the occipital region and sites where tubes, tapes and tags exist are particularly vulnerable. Pre-term neonates are at further risk due to immaturity of the corneum stratum of the skin epidermis.

Tools for assessing skin integrity

Various tools exist for assessing skin such as the Paediatric Glamorgan scale and the Braden Q scale for children. Both scales consist of several subscales: namely, mobility, activity, sensory perception, moisture, friction/shear, nutrition, and tissue perfusion/oxygenation. Each subscale is rated numerically, yielding an overall total score, which indicates the risk level for skin breakdown.

Principles of skin care

When an assessment identifies a risk as high, interventions should be implemented to reduce the risk. Preventing mechanical injury to the skin from friction and shearing forces during repositioning and transfer activity is important. A principal goal in nursing care is to reduce the external forces of pressure, shear, friction, and moisture, to prevent or treat tissue injury. Those under 8 years of age can be moved or lifted easily to prevent friction and shear. For older children, assistive devices such as lifts, trapezes, transfer boards, or mechanical lifts may be useful adjunctive devices to minimize tissue injury.

Mechanical injury from friction can be reduced with application of a barrier dressing, such as transparent films or hydrocolloids, on at-risk areas.

Interventions to reduce pressure over bony prominences are of primary importance. A turning schedule must be instituted for patients on strict bed rest. In addition to turning, heels should be suspended off the bed using pillows or heel-lift devices. A rolled-up blanket is always useful under the child's upper thighs, or the bottom of the bed can be elevated to reduce the chances of a patient sliding down in the bed. Of course, repositioning is not always an option before haemodynamic and respiratory stability is achieved.

Even with correct positioning methods, a therapeutic surface may need to be used since frequent turning may be contraindicated in unstable, critically ill children. A therapeutic surface should reduce or relieve pressure, promote blood flow to the tissues, and enable proper positioning. The therapeutic benefit of a product and its ability to maintain skin integrity will determine which type of surface will offer the best outcome. Airflow through the surface of a mattress will reduce moisture.

Mattresses/overlays have lower pressure, compared to a standard hospital mattress; examples include: an egg-crate overlay, an air-filled bed, or a special overlay which can also be beneficial in reducing shearing. A gel pillow is also useful under the occiput as a means to relieve pressure.

Superficial skin damage can also occur when adhesive products are used, although the chronically ill and critically ill are at higher risk. A skin tear or epidermal stripping is a partial thickness wound, involving tissue loss of the epidermis and possibly the dermis. Skin tears or epidermal stripping, as well as tension blisters, can easily be avoided by proper skin preparation, choice of tape, proper application and removal of tape. Skin tears resulting from adhesion can also be prevented by appropriate application and removal of tape, use of wafer skin barriers, thin hydrocolloids dressings, low-adhesion foam dressings or skin sealant under adhesives, use of porous tapes, and avoidance of unnecessary tapes.

Key points

- The maintenance of skin integrity in children is a fundamentally important aspect of nursing care and includes the assessment, prevention and treatment of pressure ulcers.
- Being mindful of the risk factors for skin breakdown, and early, regular skin assessment are essential, using the available tools for a structured approach and guide.
- Interventions that centre on the prevention of skin breakdown include risk assessment being part of care planning, being vigilant of high-risk areas of the body and clinical risk factors, regular repositioning and the use of pressure relief aids.

References

National Pressure Ulcer Advisory Panel, European Pressure Ulcer Advisory Panel and Pan Pacific Pressure Injury Alliance (2014) *Prevention and Treatment of Pressure Ulcers: Quick Reference Guide.* Ed. E. Haesler. Osborne Park, Western Australia: Cambridge Media.

Noonan, C., Quigley, S. and Curley, M. A. (2011) Using the Braden Q Scale to predict pressure ulcer risk in pediatric patients. *Journal of Pediatric Nursing*, **26**(6), 566–575.

Willock, J., Baharestani, M. M. and Anthony, D. (2009) The development of the Glamorgan Paediatric Pressure Ulcer Risk Assessment Scale. *Journal of Wound Care*, **18**(1), 17–21.

Further reading

Baharestani, M. M. and Ratliff, C. R. (2007) Pressure ulcers in neonates and children: An NPUAP White Paper. *Advances in Skin and Wound Care*, **20**(4): 208–220.

National Institute for Health and Care Excellence (2014) *Pressure Ulcers: Prevention and Management of Pressure Ulcers.* CG 179. Available at: http://www.nice.org.uk/guidance/cg179 (accessed 18 Nov. 2016).

20 Pulse oximetry

Pulse oximeter SpO$_2$ normal value, 96–100% in room air

Plethysmographic waveform. A normal signal shows a sharp waveform with a clear dicrotic notch

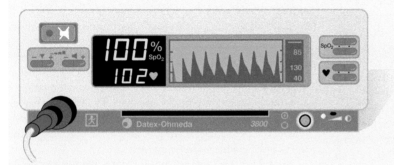

- Alarm silencer
- Upper and lower SpO$_2$ and heart rate parameter buttons
- Lead that connects to probe to patient
- Heart rate display

Position of probe

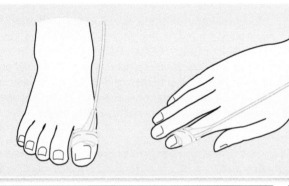

The single use adhesive probe may be sited on:

- Big toe
- Finger
- Outer aspect of foot
- Across the hand

Hinged probe

Hinged probe may be use for older children on their finger or toe

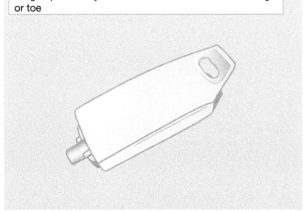

Ambulatory pulse oximeter

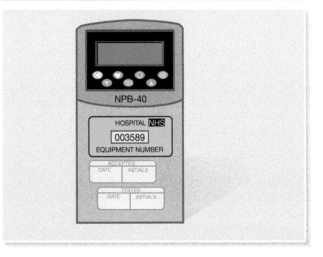

Children and Young People's Nursing Skills at a Glance, First Edition. Edited by Elizabeth Gormley-Fleming and Deborah Martin.
© 2018 John Wiley & Sons, Ltd. Published 2018 by John Wiley & Sons, Ltd.

Pulse oximetry overview

Pulse oximetry is one of the most commonly used modalities to assess and monitor the respiratory status of infants and children. It is non-invasive and may be used continuously or intermittently.

Pulse oximetry is a simple, non-invasive monitoring modality. It is used to measure the percentage of oxygen saturation (SpO_2) of haemoglobin in peripheral capillary blood. Pulse oximetry is used in the clinical setting in the hospital, the community and the home. It is one part of a patient assessment and should be used in conjunction with a complete respiratory assessment. It can be used for spot readings or for continual monitoring.

Pulse oximetry is based on two physical principles. First, the presence of a pulsatile signal generated by arterial blood which is reasonably independent of non-pulsatile arterial blood and, second, oxygenated and deoxygenated blood have different absorption spectra. Two light-emitting diodes emit red and infrared wavelengths through the tissues to a photo detector which work together. The detector measures the colour difference between the oxygenated and the deoxygenated haemoglobin during each cardiac cycle so the probe requires a constant supply of arterial blood. This information is then analysed in the calibration algorithm of the microprocessor of the pulse oximeter and the estimated arterial saturation level is displayed. This is displayed as a percentage and a waveform. A normal signal shows a sharp waveform with a clear dicrotic notch. Movement artefact and decreased perfusion will distort the waveform.

Normal value

A measurement of 95–99% in room air denotes that the haemoglobin is adequately saturated with oxygen. However, pulse oximetry cannot detect anaemia so the nurse needs to be aware of the patient's haemoglobin level, otherwise a false high reading will occur. Oximetry measures the percentage of haemoglobin that is saturated by oxygen, so if there is less haemoglobin available, then the saturated blood will have reduced oxygen-carrying capacity that is not reflected in the oximetry readings, putting the child at an increased risk of hypoxia.

Indications for use/clinical application

Pulse oximetry should be used to monitor infants and children and as a screening tool when the following conditions are present:

- the potential for respiratory failure
- respiratory illness
- haemodynamic instability
- requiring sedation or anaesthesia
- receiving oxygen therapy
- have undergone complex surgical procedures of longer than 6 hours
- under 1 year of age and are post-surgery

- during the administration of continuous respiratory depressant medication, e.g. patient-controlled analgesia
- during the transportation of infants and children intra departmental or intra hospital, who are at risk of respiratory compromise or who are already receiving oxygen therapy.

Limitations

Pulse oximetry has a number of limitations that the user needs to be aware of as these may lead to inaccurate readings. These include the following:

- When the child has low cardiac output, hypothermia or vasoconstriction, peripheral perfusion may be impaired, and as oximetry relies on detecting a pulse, it may be difficult for the sensor to detect a true signal.
- When the SpO_2 is < 70%, pulse oximetry is unreliable, due to the presence of carboxyhaemoglobin which the two wavelengths of light cannot distinguish.
- Elevated methehaemoglobin caused by either structural changes of iron in the haemoglobin or drug-induced as with local anaesthesia may lead to tissue hypoxia as the oxygen binding to the haemoglobin is inhibited.
- Smoke inhalation and carbon monoxide poisoning. The oximeter cannot distinguish between haemoglobin saturated with oxygen and that saturated with carbon monoxide.
- Motion artefact accounts for a significant number of errors and false alarms, thus shivering can cause problems with detecting saturation levels and give a false high pulse.
- The use of intravenous dyes such as methylene blue can give false low readings so nurses need to know which dye has been used and what the half-life of this is.
- The presence of oedema will lead to inaccurate measurement of the saturation level.
- Inaccurate reading will also occur in the presence of nail varnish and acrylic nails. Dried blood and dirt will also affect the accuracy of the readings and need to be removed.
- Inaccurate readings have been reported in people with dark skin and in pigmented patients. This has not been reported in jaundiced patients.
- Bright overhead lighting and external light may cause overestimation of the saturation level.

Various studies on the use of pulse oximetry as a monitoring tool for patients with sickle cell anaemia, who have acute vaso-occlusive disease, have reached different conclusions about the accuracy of the readings with up to 8% bias. Therefore, the nurse should state the child's diagnosis when reporting saturation levels.

Key points

- The correct size probe should be used.
- Alarm parameters should be set prior to commencing monitoring.
- The probe should only be secured in accordance with the manufacturer's instructions.

21 Principles of drug administration

Distraction techniques are important

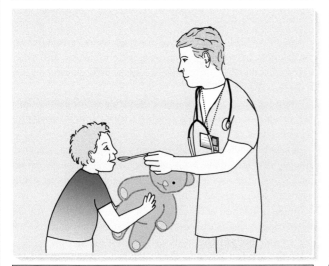

Encourage children to administer their own medication

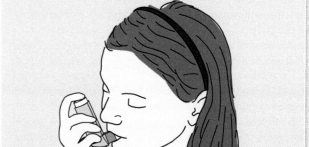

Involve parents in the administration of their child's medicine

Fundamental principles of safe drug administration

The 5 'Rs'

- Right drug
- Right dose
- Right patient
- Right route
- Right frequency

Children and Young People's Nursing Skills at a Glance, First Edition. Edited by Elizabeth Gormley-Fleming and Deborah Martin.
© 2018 John Wiley & Sons, Ltd. Published 2018 by John Wiley & Sons, Ltd.

Principles of drug administration overview

The administration of mediation is an essential aspect of nursing care. Safe practice is essential and the nurse must be aware of their professional and legal responsibilities in relation to all aspects of medication management. In relation to children's and young people's nursing practice, the nurse also needs to consider the child's developmental stage, their ability to consent to treatment and the role of parents/carers.

Key principles associated with good practice in the administration of medication are:

• The nurse should be able to demonstrate an understanding of the plan of treatment for the child.
• The prescription should be legible, unambiguous and it should be legal.
• The prescription should be checked for date prescribed, drug prescribed, dose prescribed, route prescribed, duration of treatment, any additional required information, e.g. blood levels required after second dose, and it must be signed.
• Any contraindications to the prescribed drug must be identified by the nurse and appropriate action taken.
• Allergies must be checked and noted on the prescription chart.
• The nurse needs to be aware of the effects that the medication will have on the patient and also be aware of the side effects. The child and their family should be advised accordingly so as to avoid alarm and concern.
• The paediatric formulary must be available and referred to prior to the administration of the medication.
• Medication should be prepared in a quiet area and interruption should be avoided during this period.
• The correct equipment should be collected initially.
• The nurse should check the prescription for date, time, frequency, dose, additional information and signature as part of the initial preparation process.
• The medicine container should be checked for drug name, dose, expiry date and that the content is clear and not contaminated.

• Local policy will determine the number of staff required to administer medication. Student nurses should be involved in this process.
• Consent must be obtained before you administer the medication.
• The nurse administering the medication must ensure they observe the child taking the medication.
• The medication chart should only be signed once the child has swallowed/inhaled the medication. If the child refuses the medication or is unable to receive the medication as prescribed, for whatever reason, then this must also be documented on the prescription chart.
• Involve the play therapist and employ distraction techniques as required.
• Safely dispose of all equipment used in accordance with local policy.
• Discuss any required clinical holding techniques with the child and parents before the first dose of mediation is required.
• Adhere to any additional requirements, e.g. if the medication is required to be taken on an empty stomach, then ensure this happens.
• If therapeutic serum levels are required, then ensure the child has the required blood sampling performed and that the results are available, scrutinized and acted on before any subsequent administration of the medication occurs.
• Remember the five 'Rs' of safe drug administration:
  • Right drug
  • Right dose
  • Right patient
  • Right route
  • Right frequency
• Education of the child and parents should happen early in the admission process.

Key points

• Safe practice is essential and this requires knowledge of medication, actions, interactions, contraindications along with knowing the child's treatment plan.
• Medication should be prepared in a quiet environment away from distractions.

22 Drug calculations

Nurses must be proficient in drug dose calculation

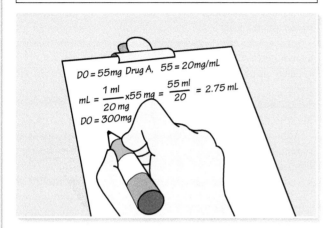

$DO = 55mg$ Drug A, $55 = 20mg/mL$

$$mL = \frac{1\ ml}{20\ mg} \times 55\ mg = \frac{55\ ml}{20} = 2.75\ mL$$

$DO = 300mg$

Calculators should be used for checking final answer

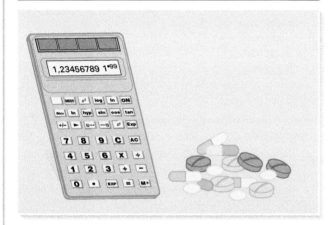

Unit convertion

1 kilogram	= 1000 grams
1 gram	= 1000 milligrams (mg)
1 mg	= 1000 micrograms (mcg)
1 mcg	= 1000 nanograms (ng)

Simple drug calculation

$$\frac{\text{What you want}}{\text{What you have}} \times \text{volume you have it in}$$

e.g. you want 100mg, you have 250mg in 5 ml. How many ml will you draw up?

$$\frac{100}{250} \times 5 = 2ml$$

Liquids should be drawn up in the correct size oral administration syringe

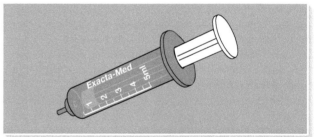

Children and Young People's Nursing Skills at a Glance, First Edition. Edited by Elizabeth Gormley-Fleming and Deborah Martin.
© 2018 John Wiley & Sons, Ltd. Published 2018 by John Wiley & Sons, Ltd.

Drug calculations overview

Competency and proficiency in the calculation of drug doses are vital for the safety of neonates, infants and children. The margin for error is significant if a decimal point is misplaced and can have life-changing and life-threatening consequences for the child. Because the population that accesses children's health care services includes both the premature neonate and the young adult, the range of doses prescribed is vast and varied. Drug calculations require basic numeracy skills.

Dose by weight

Nearly all paediatric drug doses are calculated by weight, some by body surface area and some by age. When drugs are prescribed by weight, the weight will always be in kilograms (kg). You must ensure that the child has been prescribed the correct amount of drug for their weight. Some reference books will have a suitable range, minimum to maximum dose that may be safely prescribed. It is up to the prescriber to determine which dose they are prescribing and why.

Procedure

• Local policy must be adhered to in relation to single or double checking.
• If there are two checkers, each should calculate the required drug amount independently.
• The ideal is that calculations are done in your head first, then answers may be checked with a calculator. Estimate, then guesstimate, then calculate.

There are two main formulas that are used. The first is the most commonly used:

$$\frac{\text{What you want}}{\text{What you got}} \times \frac{\text{What it is in}}{1}$$

Example: 140 mg of paracetamol is prescribed. The dose available is 250 mg in 5 ml. How much will you draw up?

$$\frac{\text{What you want is 140 mg}}{\text{What you got is 250 mg}} \times \frac{\text{What it is in is 5 ml}}{1}$$

$$\frac{140}{250} \times \frac{5}{1} = 2.8 \text{ ml}$$

The second formula is used when drugs need to be administered per kg per minute. This formula is used for intravenous drug administration of potent medication, e.g. inotropes. Errors with this calculation will lead to significant harm to the infant or child. The formula is:

$$\frac{\text{micrograms/kg/minute}}{\text{mg/ml}}$$

Example: a 7 kg baby requires 0.1 microgram/kg of epinephrine as an infusion. The solution available has 4 mg in 100 ml (40 microgram/ml).

$$\frac{0.1 \text{ (micrograms dose required)} \times 7 \text{ (weight)} \times 60 \text{ (mins)}}{40 \text{ (micrograms/ml)}}$$

$$= 1.05 \text{ ml/hr will be the volume that will be infused.}$$

The key to this calculation is to simplify, you will do this by reducing numbers to the lowest possible form, identify how many micrograms there are in a ml and convert all units to the same units where possible (e.g. mg to micrograms).

Key points
• Prior to calculating dose, check the prescription for accuracy.
• Always refer to the paediatric formulary.
• Apply the 'Estimate, guestimate, calculate' principle.
• If in any doubt about the prescription or calculation, check with the prescriber or a colleague.

23 Administration of medication

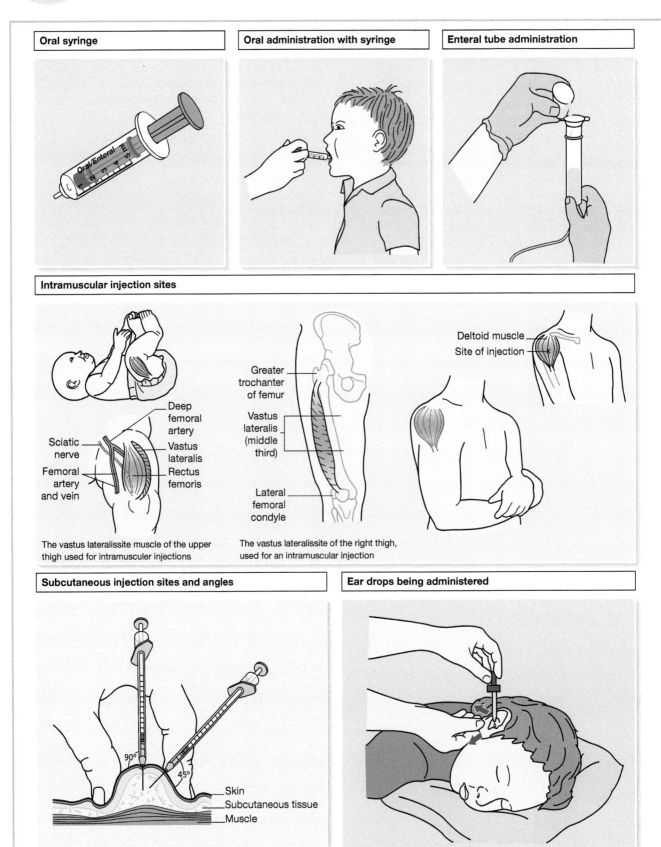

Oral syringe

Oral administration with syringe

Enteral tube administration

Intramuscular injection sites

Deep femoral artery

Sciatic nerve

Femoral artery and vein

Vastus lateralis

Rectus femoris

The vastus lateralissite muscle of the upper thigh used for intramusculer injections

Greater trochanter of femur

Vastus lateralis (middle third)

Lateral femoral condyle

The vastus lateralissite of the right thigh, used for an intramuscular injection

Deltoid muscle

Site of injection

Subcutaneous injection sites and angles

90°

45°

Skin
Subcutaneous tissue
Muscle

Ear drops being administered

Children and Young People's Nursing Skills at a Glance, First Edition. Edited by Elizabeth Gormley-Fleming and Deborah Martin.
© 2018 John Wiley & Sons, Ltd. Published 2018 by John Wiley & Sons, Ltd.

Administration of medication overview

Medication is administered through various routes: oral, via enteral tubes, subcutaneously, intramuscular, intraosseous, intravenous, inhaled, or intrathecal. The eye, ear, nose, rectum and skin are also routes through which medication can be instilled, inserted or applied. The route chosen will depend on the drug formulation available, the urgency of the treatment required, the need for the medication, local or systemic, or the speed of absorption. The preference of the child should also be a consideration. The principles of medication administration and local policy should be adhered to irrespective of the route of administration.

Oral drug administration

If the child is able to swallow, is conscious and the medication is available in an oral formulation, then this is the preferred and most convenient route. Oral medication is available as syrups, suspensions, tablets or capsules.

A sterile medication syringe or spoon should be used for liquids, and tablets should be administered in a disposable medicine pot. The syringe should be placed between the cheek and gums and the medicine gently squeezed into the child's mouth.

The infant may need to be swaddled prior to administration and incentives are beneficial when encouraging young children to take their medication.

Choice is important and should be offered.

Administration via enteral tube

This route should only be used if the child is unable to take their medication by mouth. Medications administered via this route are frequently 'off-label', so are unlicensed. It is best to discuss this route and the medication to be administered with the pharmacist.

The principles of administration of medication via enteral tubes are the same as for enteral feeding, see Chapters 38 and 39 on nasogastric/enteral feeding.

Enteric-coated medication should not be administered via the enteral tube route.

Intramuscular (IM) medication administration

This route is best avoided if possible, however, many vaccinations are administered IM. The rate of absorption is quick and this route should only be used to administer small volumes, no more than 1 ml. The preferred sites for use are:

- vastus lateralis for infants;
- deltoid for young and older children;
- ventrogluteal;
- dorsogluteal for older children only.

The gauge and length of the needle are dependent on the age of the child and the viscosity of the fluid to be administered: 25–27 gauge for infants and 22–25 for children. The injection site should be socially clean and the skin and underlying tissue should be spread to the side with a Z track technique. The needle is inserted into the skin at an angle of 90°. The plunger should be pulled back, if blood is aspirated, then discard and commence the procedure again. Otherwise inject the medication slowly, 1 ml over 10 seconds. Any faster than this will result in pain for the child. Once completed, withdraw the needle, apply gentle pressure over the site and apply a dressing if required. Dispose of waste as per local policy.

Subcutaneous administration

The subcutaneous (SC) route may be used for a single administration of medication or for infusions. The absorption rate is slower than IM and this route is suitable for small volumes. Insulin, dechelating agents, immunoglobulins, anti-coagulants are administered via the SC route. The sites that may be used for subcutaneous administration are the abdomen, upper arms, upper thighs, and buttocks. The site should be socially clean before injection. The skin should be pinched and the needle inserted at either a 45° or a 90° angle. Local policy will dictate which angle to use. The medications should be injected slowly (1 ml per 10 seconds). Withdraw the needle and dispose of as per local policy. Apply gentle pressure to the site. If the child is receiving regular SC injections, then the site should be rotated to avoid fibrosis occurring. If an infusion has been delivered SC, then an appropriate SC cannula or device should be inserted and secured as per local policy.

Administration via the eye

Administration of medication into the eye is not painful but may be uncomfortable for the child. Medication that has a local action only should be instilled or applied (ointment), e.g. antibiotics, mydriatics, to the eye.

The child should be lying down and the drop instilled into the inner cantus of the eye. Once this has been swept across the eyeball, a second drop, if prescribed, should be instilled. Ointment should be instilled inside the lower lid. The lower lid should be pulled back and a line of ointment applied. Care should be taken when administering eye drops or ointment not to touch the child with the dropper or nozzle of the ointment tube as this will contaminate the medication. If both eyes are being treated, then there should be two tubes of ointment or eye drops.

Administration via the ear

Locally acting medication may be instilled into the ear, e.g. antibiotics, steroids. It may be difficult to gain the cooperation of the very young child. The child should lie with the ear to be treated facing upright. Having prepared and checked the medication, pull the pinna up and back and gently insert the prescribed number of drops directly into the ear canal. Massage the tragus of the ear and ask the child to lie still for 5 minutes. If the child is less than 3 years of age, pull the pinna down and back in order to access the ear canal.

Per rectum medication administration

Privacy and dignity must be maintained when administering medication per rectum. This route should only be used when it is not possible to administer the medication through any other route, e.g. the child is vomiting and has not got an intravenous cannula in situ or it is required for local treatment.

The child should be asked to void urine first and then once returned to their bed, asked to lie on their left side with their legs flexed. If possible, ask the child to breathe deeply as this will help to relax them. Lubricate the suppository or enema tube, insert the rounded end of the suppository first for the nozzle. Remove the nozzle once the liquid has been inserted. Hold the buttocks gently together as this will help the child retain the medication. A toilet or commode should be nearby for the child to access if required.

Key points
- Where appropriate, offer the child a choice, e.g. spoon or a medicine syringe, liquid or tablet.
- With injections, rotate the site if frequent administrations are required.

24 Inhaled drug administration

Metered dose inhaler components

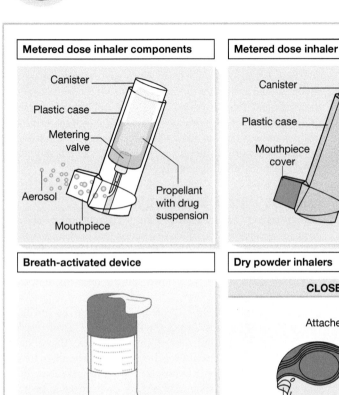

Canister
Plastic case
Metering valve
Aerosol
Mouthpiece
Propellant with drug suspension

Metered dose inhaler

Canister
Plastic case
Mouthpiece cover
Base

Spacer device

AeroChamber

Breath-activated device

Dry powder inhalers

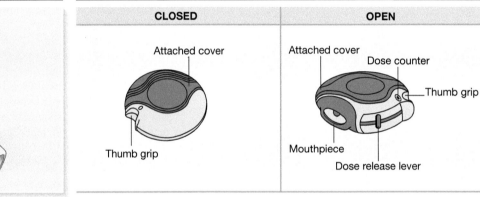

CLOSED	OPEN
Attached cover	Attached cover
Thumb grip	Dose counter
	Thumb grip
	Mouthpiece
	Dose release lever

Child using spacer device

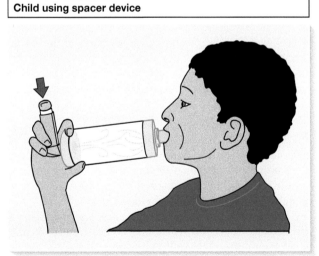

Infant using spacer device

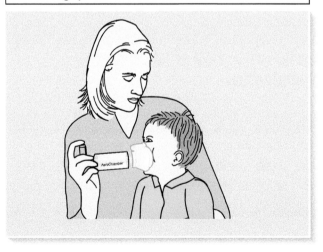

AeroChamber

Children and Young People's Nursing Skills at a Glance, First Edition. Edited by Elizabeth Gormley-Fleming and Deborah Martin.
© 2018 John Wiley & Sons, Ltd. Published 2018 by John Wiley & Sons, Ltd.

Inhaled drug administration overview

The inhaled route of drug administration is widely accepted as being the optimal way of giving drugs, such as corticosteroids and bronchodilators for the treatment of patients with airflow obstruction, e.g. asthma, cystic fibrosis. The inhaled route allows relatively small doses of drugs to be delivered to produce high concentrations in the airway but minimizes absorption into the systemic circulation. This will then reduce the incidence of side effects from the medication. However, a proper inhaler technique with inhaler devices is essential to achieve the correct dose.

Devices

There are various devices available: metered dose inhalers (MDIs), MDIs with spacers, dry powder inhalers (DPIs) and breath-activated MDIs (BA-MDI).

Metered dose inhalers (MDIs)

This is the standard mechanism for delivering drugs to small airways. It is essential that the patient/parent/carer is educated in the use of the device and that competence is checked. Adequate coordination is required.

• To use: shake inhaler to ensure inhaler is primed.
• Ask the child to exhale, place the mouthpiece in the child's mouth. The child should commence breathing in as soon as the inhaler is pressed downwards to release the medication. They should continue to breathe in slowly and hold their breath for 10 seconds. If a second dose is required, the child should wait 30 seconds before this is administered.

Breath-activated MDIs (BA-MDIs)

These devices allow the patient to prime the inhaler first and then when the patient takes a breath, the inhaler is activated. It avoids the need to coordinate breathing with release of the inhaler. It is useful for older children if they are able to use the device effectively.

Spacer devices

Spacer devices slow down the particles and make coordination of activation and inhalation much less critical. They are useful for infants and children with poor inhaler technique. The main advantage is that they increase the proportion of dose delivered to the airways while reducing the proportion absorbed in the body. Inhalation from the spacer device should follow activation as soon as possible as the drug aerosol is very short-lived. The dose should be administered as a single actuation with tidal breathing for 10–20 seconds or five breaths.

Corticosteroid and bronchodilator therapy should be delivered by a pressurized MDI and spacer device (with a facemask if necessary) to children under 5 years. For children aged 5–15 years, corticosteroid therapy should be delivered by a MDI and spacer device. Spacers should be replaced annually or as the child grows and the spacer no longer is fit for their size. Cleaning should be carried out in accordance with manufacturer's instructions.

Dry powder inhalers (DPIs)

These are small and portable, like MDIs, but require less coordination. The drug delivery to the lungs is dependent upon the patient's peak inhaled flow rate. These may be useful for children over 5 years who are unwilling or unable to use a MDI with a spacer device.

The technique is the same as for MDIs but the number of doses available should be checked on the counter, then hold it horizontally, open the casing and push the level until it clicks. The dose is then ready for administration.

Key points
• The cooperation of the child is required.
• Compliance with treatment is important so detailed discussion is essential in relation to the treatment plan.
• Incorrect technique is common and will result in inadequate dose administration.
• Refresh the technique of child/parents/carers on a regular basis.
• Be satisfied that parents/carers know when the inhaler device is running low.

25 Intranasal diamorphine

Equipment used to administer intranasal diamorphine

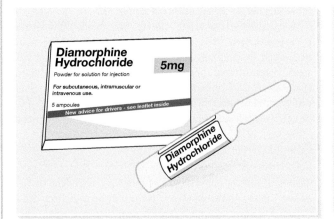

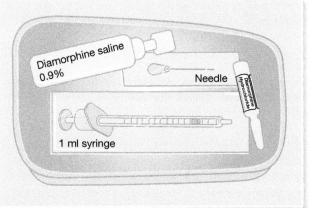

Contraindications

- Children under 1 year unless directed by a senior doctor

- Children over 60 kgs

- Head injury or reduced conscious level

- Blocked nose, e.g. trauma to nose

- Respiratory compromise

- Contraindications to opiates

Weight calculation method
Source: Advanced Life Support Group (2015). Reproduced with permission of John Wiley & Sons

- Child 0–1 year = (Age in months/2) + 4
  e.g. 8-months-old child: 8/2 = 4 + 4 = 8 kgs

- Child 5–5 years = (Age x 2) + 8
  e.g. 2-year-old child: 2 x 2 + 8 = 12 kgs

- Child 6–12 years = (Age x 3) + 7
  e.g. 10-year-old child: 10 x 3 + 7 = 37 kgs

Calculation table for Intranasal Diamorphine
Always give 0.2 mls

Child's weight (kgs)	Volume of saline to be added (mls)
10	2
15	1.3
20	1
25	0.8
30	0.7
35	0.6
40	0.5
45	0.45
50	0.4
55	0.35
60	0.3

Children and Young People's Nursing Skills at a Glance, First Edition. Edited by Elizabeth Gormley-Fleming and Deborah Martin.
© 2018 John Wiley & Sons, Ltd. Published 2018 by John Wiley & Sons, Ltd.

Intranasal diamorphine overview

Intranasal diamorphine is described in much of the literature as a safe and effective analgesia which can be used for children with moderate and severe pain. In the emergency setting and on the wards, the use of intranasal diamorphine has increased as it is non-invasive with a rapid analgesic effect, few side effects and a rapid excretion of the medication, so that it can be used while more longer-acting medication is being prepared or for a short-term painful procedure such as applying a plaster of Paris to a fractured radius and ulna.

Diamorphine is a controlled drug and is subject to the Controlled Drugs Act 2006. It is a type of medicine called an opioid painkiller. It is also known as 'medical heroin'. Opioids treat pain by mimicking the action of naturally occurring pain-reducing chemicals called endorphins, which are present in the brain and spinal cord and reduce pain by combining with opioid receptors. Diamorphine can be administered via a syringe or via a new atomizer product which has just been licensed. In this chapter we will discuss the syringe method as, due to the high cost of the atomizer, as yet it is not used in all hospitals.

Equipment

- 1 vial of diamorphine (10 mg)
- saline for injection
- 1 ml syringe
- 1 needle
- 2 nurses
- saturation monitoring equipment.

Patients

- Children with moderate to severe pain (or mild pain where other analgesia is difficult to administer)
- Children over 1 year or 10 kg
- Can be used in children under 10 kg but must be under the supervision of a senior doctor.

The nurse/practitioner

- The nurse must have had training in the use of intranasal diamorphine.
- The drug must be prescribed by a doctor or using a patient group directive if available.
- Two nurses must prepare and administer the medication as it is a controlled drug.

Contraindications

- Calculations: weigh child if possible or use calculation methods as per *Advanced Paediatric Life Support Manual.*
- Dilute diamorphine with saline.
- Always give 0.2 ml into one nostril. This will give the child 100 micrograms/kg.

Administration

- The preparation has an unpleasant taste and often giving paracetamol directly after administering the medication helps to take the taste away. A small amount of fluid can be given but the child may require surgery, so reducing the amount of fluid ingested should be considered.

- Place the child in an upright position. Explain the procedure to the child, explaining that it does not taste nice and offer a solution to the child for this.
- Older children can be encouraged to sniff gently once the medication has been squirted into the nostril.
- Younger children can sit on the knee of the carer, who can tip the child back slightly to allow sufficient time for the medication to be absorbed by the mucosa.
- The medication starts to work in a few minutes although this can vary from child to child.
- Although side effects are rare, where possible, the child should have oxygen saturation monitoring on site. In reality, a child requiring this medication is frequently too agitated to tolerate monitoring and the practitioner should stay with the child, monitoring their colour or any signs of respiratory distress (heart rate, respiratory rate, saturations). This should be done for 30 minutes.
- Assess level of consciousness.

Additional points

- Diamorphine works quickly but further analgesia is likely to be required.
- No other opioid should be given for 20 minutes after administration of diamorphine.
- Apply local anaesthetic if the child is likely to require cannulation.
- Diamorphine can be repeated after 30 minutes if required.
- Children tend to become calm and relaxed post administration.
- Reassess pain every 15 minutes until the child is pain-free.

Documentation

- Two registered nurses must sign the Controlled Drugs book, including indicating the unused medication disposal.
- Two registered nurses are required to sign the drug chart.
- Document consent from carer and child.
- List nostril used.
- List pain score.

Intranasal diamorphine is an effective and reasonably non-invasive analgesia. It is used frequently in the emergency department but its use could be much wider as it helps children cope with a variety of unpleasant procedures.

Key points
- The nasal mucosa should be intact and, if not, this route should be avoided.
- The procedure is pain-free.
- Distraction needs should be considered.

Reference

Advanced Life Support Group (2015) *Advanced Paediatric Life Support Manual: A Practical Approach to Emergencies.* 6th edition. Wiley Blackwell, Oxford.

Further reading

College of Emergency Medicine, Clinical Effectiveness Committee (2010) *Guidelines for the Management of Pain in Children.* CEM, London.

The Controlled Drugs (Supervision of Management and Use) Regulation (2006) No. 38.

26 Intravenous fluid administration

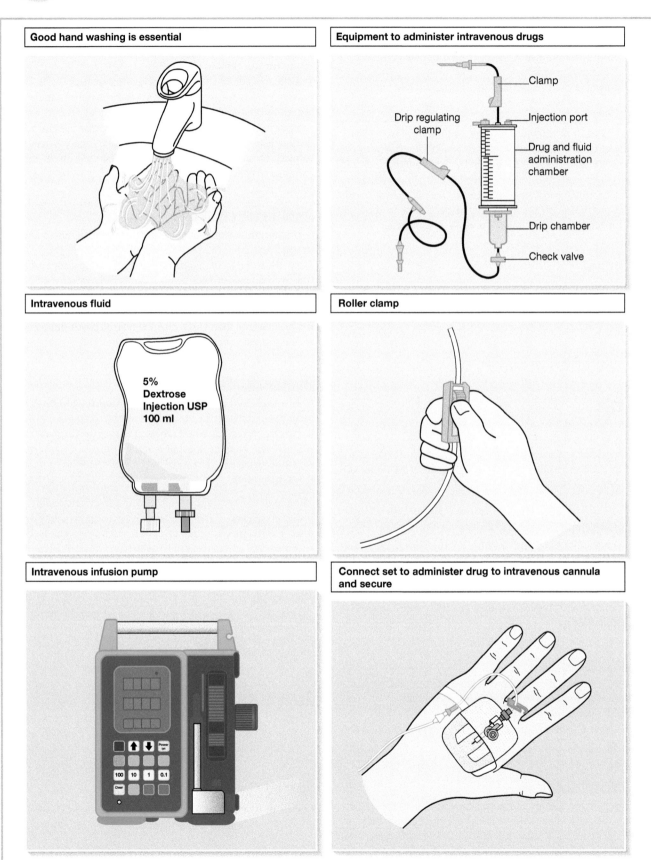

Good hand washing is essential

Equipment to administer intravenous drugs

Clamp

Drip regulating clamp

Injection port

Drug and fluid administration chamber

Drip chamber

Check valve

Intravenous fluid

5% Dextrose Injection USP 100 ml

Roller clamp

Intravenous infusion pump

Connect set to administer drug to intravenous cannula and secure

Children and Young People's Nursing Skills at a Glance, First Edition. Edited by Elizabeth Gormley-Fleming and Deborah Martin.
© 2018 John Wiley & Sons, Ltd. Published 2018 by John Wiley & Sons, Ltd.

Intravenous fluid administration overview

The changing of the intravenous fluid bag and administration sets must be done following the aseptic non-touch technique (ANTT) and as per local policy. If the correct procedure is not followed, then the child is at risk of developing sepsis or possible air embolus. Any fluids or drugs that are to be added to the intravenous fluids must be compatible.

Equipment
- Prescription chart
- Administration set
- Intravenous fluid
- Sterile field
- Single patient alcohol wipe
- Gloves
- Apron

Procedure
- Assemble equipment.
- Wash and dry hands thoroughly.
- Check intravenous fluid as per local policy against the prescription chart.
- Observe the outer wrapper, making sure it is intact.
- Check the fluids expiry date, colour, clarity and for the presence of any particles.
- Check the outer wrapper of the administration set to make sure it is intact and that it has not expired.
- Open administration set and close the roller clamp.
- Open the intravenous fluid bag and expose the port by removing the protective cover.
- Remove the protective cover on the administration set's spike and using ANTT, insert into the intravenous fluid bag.
- Hang the intravenous fluid bag on a drip stand.
- Squeeze the drip chamber of the administration set until it is half-full.

- Slowly open the roller clamp and prime the administration set until the fluid reaches the end of the line, following the manufacturer's instructions. This should expel the air from the line but visually inspect the line for the presence of any air. If air is present, then open the roller clamp to allow more fluid through the line, expelling any remaining air.
- Close the roller clamp.
- If using a burette, then fill approximately 30 ml of fluids into the burette and close the fluid-fill clamp before opening the roller clamp to prime the line.
- Insert the administration set into the appropriate infusion pump.
- Check the patient's identity.
- When using a needleless device, e.g. Smartsite,™ decontaminate as per local policy or remove Luer Lok™.
- Ensure the patency of the intravenous cannula prior to connecting the intravenous infusion by flushing with 0.9% normal saline as prescribed.
- Connect the administration set to the intravenous cannula.
- Secure the administration set as required.
- Set the infusion rate and the other parameters as prescribed.
- Open the roller clamp and commence the infusion.
- Document all the required details, batch number, expiry date, time infusion commenced, name of first and second checker on prescription chart.
- Document the date and time of when the administration set was changed in the child's care records along with the serial number of the pump being used.
- Remove the apron and gloves and dispose of all waste.
- Commence/maintain fluid balance chart.
- Wash and dry hands thoroughly.

Key points
- Always allow intravenous fluid to flow slowly through the line so as to avoid 'air bubbles'.
- Place the roller clamp near the intravenous fluid bag so the nurse can have easy access to this in the event of pump malfunction.
- Label the line with the date and time that it was first used.

27 Spirometry

Spirometry

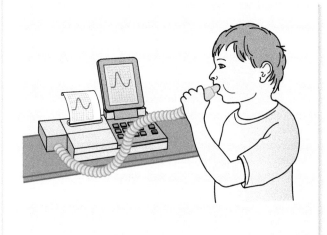

Respiratory system

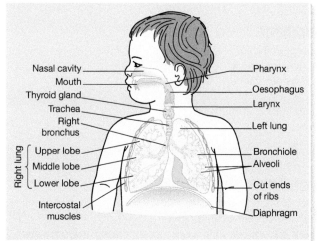

Nose clip in situ

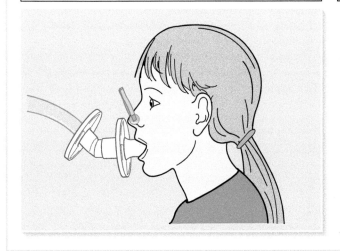

Lung function results

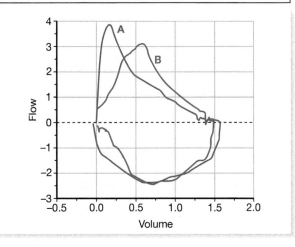

Children and Young People's Nursing Skills at a Glance, First Edition. Edited by Elizabeth Gormley-Fleming and Deborah Martin.
© 2018 John Wiley & Sons, Ltd. Published 2018 by John Wiley & Sons, Ltd.

Spirometry overview

Spirometry is the most commonly used lung function test in the management of respiratory disease. It is an effective tool in diagnosing lung disease and measuring the response to treatment in a variety of patients. Respiratory disorders can cause changes within the lungs and airways, Spirometry tests are valuable in detecting abnormalities and therefore changes within the lungs. To understand the procedure, it is useful to understand the anatomy and physiology of the respiratory system. Spirometry usually identifies one of four patterns:

- normal;
- an obstructive pattern (asthma, COPD);
- a restrictive pattern (fibrosing alveolitis, scoliosis);
- a combined obstructive/restrictive pattern.

There are numerous different spirometer machines on the market. Some machines will automatically calculate the predicted values and others require manual calculations done by the practitioner. Spirometry is a good tool for measuring the effectiveness of inhaled and exhaled breath. A dynamic lung function test will measure the amount (volume) and speed (flow) of the air during forced inspiratory and expiratory breath. A spirometer measures a variety of parameters. The most commonly used tests are shown below.

- *Forced vital capacity (FVC)*: This is the maximum volume of air which can be expelled from the lungs during a long forced and complete expiration (maximum out-breath) from a position of full inspiration (maximum in-breath).
- *Forced expiratory volume in 1 second (FEV1)*: This measures the maximum volume of air which can be expelled from the lungs in the first second of forced expiration (out-breath).
- *Peak expiratory flow (PEF)*: This is the maximum flow achieved from a short forced expiration (out-breath). It is commonly called a peak flow (see Chapter 28).
- *Forced vital capacity/Forced expiratory volume in 1 second (FVC/FEV1)*: The ratio between FVC and FEV1 expressed as a percentage.

Technique

All equipment must be clean and a bacterial filter used for each patient to avoid cross-contamination of equipment. First, prepare the patient and spirometer for the test. It is essential to obtain the patient's consent and ensure that they are aware of the procedure and its purpose. Record the patient's gender, most recent height and weight and ethnicity correctly into the spirometer. (Normal values for lung volumes are based on these aspects.) The British Thoracic Society (BTS) guidelines recommend that the patient is sitting during the test as forced expiratory manoeuvres may make the patient feel faint.

Procedure

To obtain a forced spirometry test:

- Ensure the patient is wearing nose clips to prevent air leaks from the nose.
- Ask the patient to breathe in as fully as possible.
- Ensure they seal lips and teeth tightly around the mouthpiece.
- Make them blow out forcibly, as hard and as fast as possible until all air is expelled from lungs.
- Patients are advised not to lean forward during the test.

A minimum of three attempts is required and the result reported should be the highest value achieved from three successful attempts. Consider the patient's capability and age to accurately perform the test. The BTS guidelines recommend health care professionals assess technique on an individual basis and only to begin teaching spirometry technique for children above 5 years of age.

Interpreting the results

The NICE guidelines recommend that all practitioners should be competent in the interpretation of the results of spirometry and should have received appropriate training and keep their skills up to date.

Lung function results are reported in absolute values in litres. Using the best of the three consistent readings, identify the predicted values according to weight, height and gender. Compare the reading from the patient with the prediction chart. Some machines interpret the results in data format automatically.

If airways are narrowed, then the amount of air which is expelled (breathed out) is reduced. Therefore, the FEV1 and the ratio of FEV1/FVC will be lower than normal/predicted. Lung volumes of 80–120% of predicted values are considered to be within normal limits.

Key points
- Technique is important, as otherwise, results will be inaccurate.
- Mouthpieces must be single use.

28 Peak expiratory flow

Peak flow chart: children both boys and girls
Source: Redrawn from Godfrey et al. (1970)

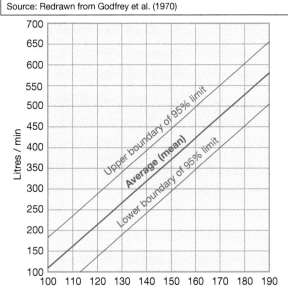

Graphic representation of how to calculate expected peak flow value

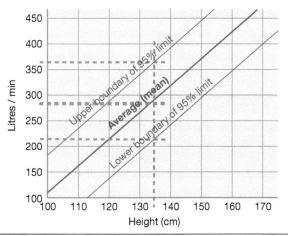

Peak flow meter

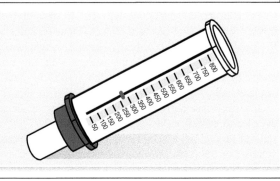

Child using peak flow meter

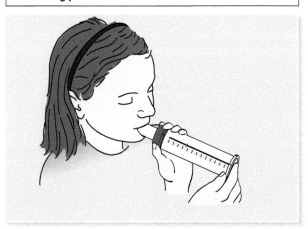

How to use a peak flow meter

1. Set to 0	2. Breathe in	3. Blow as hard as you can	4. Repeat three times and record the highest reading

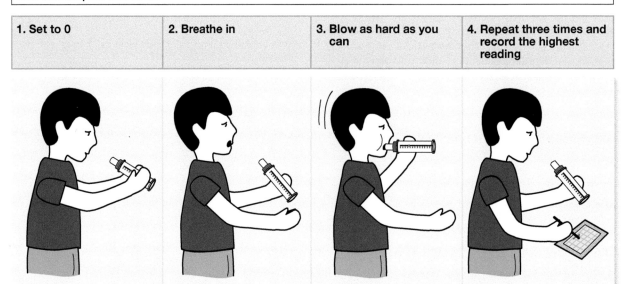

Children and Young People's Nursing Skills at a Glance, First Edition. Edited by Elizabeth Gormley-Fleming and Deborah Martin.
© 2018 John Wiley & Sons, Ltd. Published 2018 by John Wiley & Sons, Ltd.

Peak expiratory flow overview

Peak expiratory flow measures the maximum rate of air blown out of the lungs on expiration. A small portable hand-held device is used with a mouthpiece. The measurement obtained indicates the degree of airway narrowing and obstruction. It is used in patients with asthma to aid diagnosis and monitor the effectiveness of treatment, and determine if the asthma is worsening.

To aid diagnosis, patients may be asked to keep a diary of peak flow measurements twice daily for a week. If the airways are narrowed, the speed at which the air leaves the lungs is reduced, therefore the peak flow would be lower than expected. This is typically in the morning or if the patient is unwell.

Regular peak flow readings are used in addition to a review of asthma symptoms, and they are used as a self-management tool. Readings are taken before and after treatment to open up the airways to monitor its effectiveness. Peak flow readings should improve if the treatment plan is working as the airways are less constricted.

Procedure

• The child and parents should be given information about the procedure and that it may induce coughing or wheezing.
• The marker on the peak flow meter should be reset to zero.
• The child should be standing upright.
• The child should take a deep breath, seal the lips around the mouthpiece and blow out as hard and as fast as possible.
• The marker reading should be noted on the meter.
• Reset the marker and repeat this up to three times. The highest of the three values should be recorded.

The correct technique must be observed in order to reduce misleading results. The accuracy of peak flow can be affected by:

• the behaviour of children who have never performed a peak flow before or younger children who are unable to follow the directions of use (usually under 5 years of age);

• a poor seal around the mouthpiece or the tongue blocking the mouthpiece;
• the child not blowing as hard as possible;
• the use of different peak flow meters.

How is peak flow recorded and what are normal readings?

Peak flow is recorded in litres per minute (L/min). It is routinely documented on a graph which predicts normal values based upon a child's sex, height and age.

The calculation for children below 15 years of age is:

$$\text{Peak expiratory flow} = 455 \times (\text{height}/100) - 332$$

• Green (Safe zone) – Peak flow reading is normal or near the personal best, 80–100%.
• Yellow (Caution zone) – Peak flow is lower than child's personal best, 50–80%. The airways are inflamed, moderate asthma exacerbation.
• Red (Danger zone) – Peak flow is significantly lower than the child's personal best, less than 50%. Airway is narrowing, which occurs during acute severe asthma.

However, always assess the patient's best peak flow reading in addition to the predicted peak flow value, taking into consideration the patient's technique.

Key points
• This is a technique that the child needs to develop and it is best practised when the child is well.
• It is important to note the child's personal best value as it may be outside of the normal expected range.

Reference

Godfrey, S., Kamburoff, P. L., and Nairn, J. N. (1970) Spirometry, lung volumes and airway resistance in normal children aged 5–18 years. *British Journal of Diseases of the Chest*, 64: 15–24.

29 Arterial blood gas sampling

Common causes of blood gas disturbance

Metabolic acidosis pH 7.35	Severe gastroenteritis Diabetic ketoacidosis Shock-hypovolemic, cardiogenic Birth asphyxia
Metabolic alkalosis pH >7.45	Pyloric stenosis Diuretics Excessive naso-gastric tube losses
Respiratory acidosis	Respiratory failure due to illness or any other cause e.g. asthma, inadequate mechanical ventilation, CNS depression
Respiratory alkalosis	Hyperventilation Excessive mechanical ventilation

Location of radial artery

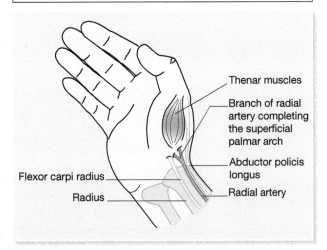

Thenar muscles
Branch of radial artery completing the superficial palmar arch
Abductor policis longus
Radial artery
Flexor carpi radius
Radius

Blood gas analyser

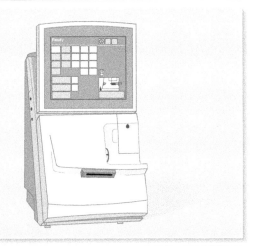

Location of femoral artery

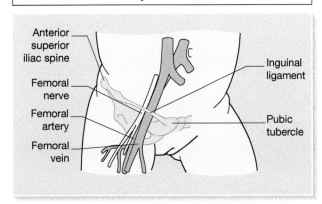

Anterior superior iliac spine
Femoral nerve
Femoral artery
Femoral vein
Inguinal ligament
Pubic tubercle

Blood gas values

Normal range for acid base and blood gas measurement

Arterial pH 7.36–7.42

Arterial PaCO$_2$ 4.7–5.5 kPa

Arterial PaO$_2$ 11–14 kPa (8–10 kPa in neonates)

Arterial or venous bicarbonate 17–27 mmols/L

Base excess >0–2 mmols/l

Children and Young People's Nursing Skills at a Glance, First Edition. Edited by Elizabeth Gormley-Fleming and Deborah Martin.
© 2018 John Wiley & Sons, Ltd. Published 2018 by John Wiley & Sons, Ltd.

Arterial blood gas sampling overview

Acid base disturbances are indicators of serious underlying pathology. An arterial blood gas (ABG) analysis can provide vital information for a paediatric clinical assessment and aid in decision-making, especially in children suffering from respiratory distress. It is an essential tool in diagnosing and managing a child's oxygenation status and acid base balance. A blood gas analysis also provides other vital information, such as blood sugar, haemoglobin, bilirubin, and electrolyte values, such as sodium, potassium, calcium and chloride levels. Blood gas sampling can be taken from an artery, a vein or a capillary. However, arterial sampling is considered to be more accurate.

Procedure

There are two ways to obtain an ABG sample:

1 an aseptic direct arterial puncture with a heparinized syringe, using local anaesthesia. The syringe is heparinized to stop clotting.
2 an indwelling arterial cannula. The cannula should be situated in a radial artery by preference; however, the umbilical, brachial or femoral can be used.

Equipment

- A 25 G needle or a 25 G butterfly needle.
- A 2 ml syringe with heparin.
- A cap for the syringe.
- A local anaesthetic (plus needle and syringe for administering it).
- Alcohol gel.
- Gauze.
- Gloves and apron.
- A sharps bin.
- A blood gas analyser.

How to collect a blood gas sample from an artery

- Explain the need for blood gas to the child and the parent, if possible, and obtain consent.
- Wash your hands and wear personal protection equipment such as apron and gloves.
- Position the child's arm with wrist extended.
- Locate the radial artery by checking the pulsation.
- Attach the needle to the heparinized syringe, and a local anaesthetic to be used prior to the procedure if it is non-emergency.
- Insert the needle 30 degrees to the skin where maximum pulsation is felt.
- Advance the needle until arterial blood rushes into the syringe.
- Remove the needle once a sufficient sample has been obtained.
- Press firmly over the puncture site for 5 minutes with gauze.
- Discard the needle in the sharps bin and place a bung over the syringe taking careful consideration to remove any air from the syringe.
- Immediately analyse the sample in a blood gas machine.
- Dispose of all the waste.
- Wash your hands and record the results.
- This procedure is usually undertaken by a doctor.

Blood gas interpretation

Acid-base evaluation requires a focus on three of the reported components: pH, $PaCO_2$ and HCO_3.

- *pH (potential hydrogen)* = the pH determines the acidity or alkalinity of the blood. The normal pH of the blood is between 7.35 and 7.45.
  - Acidosis = pH less than 7.35;
  - Alkalosis = pH more than 7.45.
- $PaCO_2$ = this relates to the partial pressure of carbon dioxide (CO_2) dissolved in plasma. This is the respiratory component of the blood gas. The normal $PaCO_2$ values are 5–6 kPa or 38–42 mmHg. An increase in $PaCO_2$ will therefore indicate that, for some reason, carbon dioxide is not being eliminated.
- HCO_3 = bicarbonate is also known as a 'base' and is present in blood within a range of 22–28 mmol/l. This is the renal component of the blood gas.

If the pH and $PaCO_2$ are indeed moving in *opposite directions*, then the problem is primarily *respiratory* in nature. If the pH and HCO_3 are moving *in the same direction*, then the problem is primarily *metabolic* in nature.

The arterial PaO_2 normal range is 11–14 kPa (8–10 kPa in neonates). A high reading will likely be an indicator of respiratory alkalosis and a low reading will indicate respiratory acidosis.

A useful acronym to remember is ROME:

Respiratory
Opposite
Metabolic
Equal

Examples of acid base disturbances are:

- *Respiratory acidosis*: a pH less than 7.35 with a $PaCO_2$ greater than 45 mmHg. This occurs when there is inadequate ventilation and CO_2 production is greater than the CO_2 elimination. The common causes are airway obstruction, respiratory depression due to drugs, head injury and lung diseases.
- *Respiratory alkalosis*: a pH greater than 7.45 with a $PaCO_2$ less than 38 mmHg. This occurs with hyperventilation. Factors such as pain, anxiety, fear and medications such as respiratory stimulants can cause this.
- *Metabolic acidosis*: a bicarbonate level of less than 22 mEq/l with a pH of less than 7.35. Etiologies are loss of bicarbonate due to GIT losses or chronic renal disease, addition of inorganic acids such as diabetic ketoacidosis, lactic acidosis due to tissue hypoxia, salicylate, decreased acid excretion in renal failure and toxins.
- *Metabolic alkalosis*: a bicarbonate level greater than 28 mEq/l with a pH greater than 7.45. Usually associated with an excess of a base or loss of an acid. Examples are loss of gastric acid due to vomiting and diuretic therapy.

Key points

- Careful consideration has to be given when interpreting the blood gas values. Emphasis has to be placed on the child's vital signs such as temperature and oxygenation during sampling.
- Be aware of the different units used in different settings such as kPa and mmHg.
- If a child requires frequent arterial sampling, then it would be ideal to have an indwelling arterial catheter in place to avoid further distress.
- Only professionals who are competent in performing the arterial sampling should carry out the procedure.

30 Oxygen administration

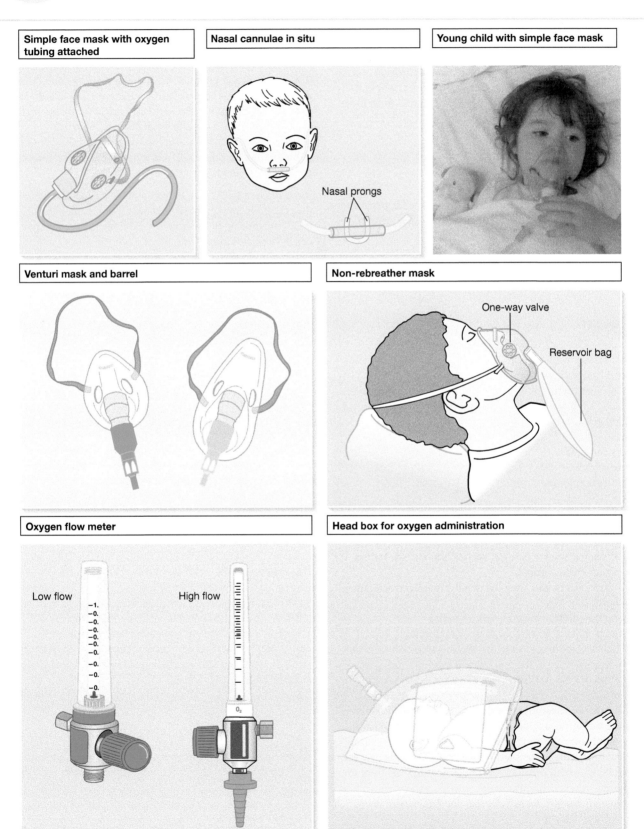

Simple face mask with oxygen tubing attached

Nasal cannulae in situ

Nasal prongs

Young child with simple face mask

Venturi mask and barrel

Non-rebreather mask

One-way valve

Reservoir bag

Oxygen flow meter

Low flow

High flow

O_2

Head box for oxygen administration

Children and Young People's Nursing Skills at a Glance, First Edition. Edited by Elizabeth Gormley-Fleming and Deborah Martin.
© 2018 John Wiley & Sons, Ltd. Published 2018 by John Wiley & Sons, Ltd.

Oxygen administration overview

Oxygen is frequently administered to infants and children in the hospital setting as part of the management of acute and chronic illness. Safe practice is paramount as inappropriate use of oxygen can be hazardous to the infant/child, e.g. in certain cardiac conditions. A complete systematic assessment must be undertaken to identify the child's clinical condition prior to the administration of oxygen. The exception to this would be in an emergency situation where high flow oxygen is usually administered initially.

Administration of oxygen

Oxygen is administered through:

- nasal cannulae;
- a simple mask;
- a Venturi mask;
- a non-rebreather mask;
- a head box.

Equipment

- Oxygen-cylinder supply or central supply.
- Oxygen flow meter.
- Appropriate oxygen delivery device (nasal cannulae, face mask).
- Oxygen saturation monitor and correct size of probe.
- Oxygen tubing.
- Elephant tubing for head box.
- Oxygen analyser for head box.
- Consider humidification.
- Paediatric Early Warning Scoring chart.

Procedure

- Wash your hands
- Place correct size of administration device in nostrils/over child's nose and mouth.
- Secure as per local policy.
- Connect oxygen tubing to oxygen flow meter.
- Turn on oxygen supply to the prescribed flow rate.
- Monitor and record the child's oxygen saturation level, heart rate, and respiratory rate.
- Note the work of breathing and the child's colour.

All children who require oxygen will need ongoing assessment and monitoring of their condition. The amount of oxygen delivered and the device used should be recorded, as should the effectiveness of the treatment.

The amount of oxygen to be administered must be prescribed. Oxygen should be weaned and discontinued as soon as possible. Increasing oxygen requirements indicate a deteriorating infant/child.

Nasal cannulae

Nasal cannulae should only be used to deliver a flow rate of 0–2 L per minute. If a higher flow rate is required, then an alternate device will be required. Humidification is not required.

Nasal cannulae consist of two soft prongs that arise from the oxygen tubing. The prongs are placed in the infant's/child's nostrils with the prongs pointing downwards. This will avoid undue pressure on the nasal mucosa. When using with infants, ensure the prongs do not completely block the nostril as infants are obligatory nasal breathers.

The oxygen tubing may be secured with an appropriate dressing. When used with an older child, they may be secured at the back of the child's head, sitting over the pinna of the ear.

Ideal for low flow oxygen delivery, the prongs may become blocked with secretions and irritate the nasal mucosa by drying it out.

Simple face mask

A simple face mask can be used to deliver oxygen of various concentrations by adjusting the flow rate via the flow meter. A flow rate of > 4l/min is required to prevent the rebreathing of exhaled carbon dioxide.

Face masks come in various sizes and should fit comfortably over the child's nose and mouth. A good seal is important. Not all children can tolerate a face mask so careful planning and explanations are required. The child may not want the mask on their face. Face masks are not intended for long-term use. A simple face mask will deliver a maximum fractional inspired oxygen concentration (FiO2) of 50%.

Venturi mask

A Venturi mask permits the delivery of various concentrations of oxygen: 24%, 28%, 35%, 40% and 60% depending on the colour of the barrel chosen and the oxygen flow rate.

One side of the coloured barrel indicates the percentage of oxygen and the other side shows then number of litres to set the flow meter. To alter the amount of oxygen, the barrel needs to be changed.

Non-rebreather mask

The use of a non-rebreather mask with a reservoir bag can enable the inspired oxygen concentration level of 99% with a high flow of 10–15 L/min. The high flow will prevent carbon dioxide from being inhaled. It should not be used if a high flow rate cannot be maintained. The high flow will keep the reservoir bag inflated and the bag should be inflated prior to use. A non-rebreather mask is for short-term emergency use only.

Head box

Head boxes are only suitable for infants of less than 9 months of age who require high flow oxygen delivery, and it can deliver a FiO2 of > 95%.

The head box is placed over the infant's head with their shoulders outside. Elephant tubing is required to deliver the humidified oxygen to the infant.

An oxygen analyser is required and this should be calibrated to measure the percentage of oxygen being administered. This needs to be placed as close to the infant's airway as possible. Gas escape routes should not be covered as a build-up of carbon dioxide will occur. The flow rate will need to be maintained to prevent carbon dioxide from building up.

The head box will mist up when humidification is being used, so monitoring the infant's temperature is important – cold stress or pyrexia is most likely. Have an alternate oxygen administration device ready as the removal of head box will lead to a sudden decrease of oxygen concentration.

Consider placing a familiar toy in the infant's line of sight.

Key points
- A secure, tight-fitting device is required for the effective delivery of oxygen.
- Oxygen should not be prescribed except in an emergency.
- Increasing oxygen requirements indicate a deteriorating infant/child.
- Regular monitoring of vital signs is essential.

31 Suctioning

Suction catheter

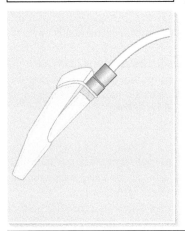

Measuring length of suction catheter

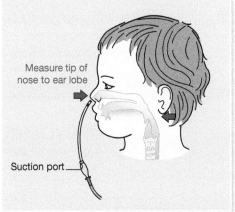

Measure tip of nose to ear lobe

Suction port

Yankeur suction catheter

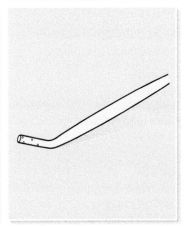

Portable suction unit

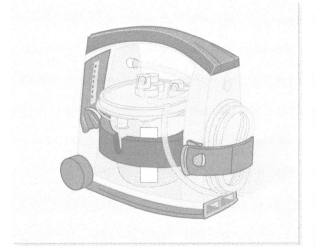

Wall-mounted suction unit

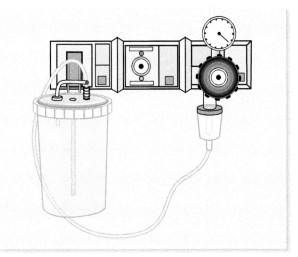

Head holding position to enable safe suctioning procedure

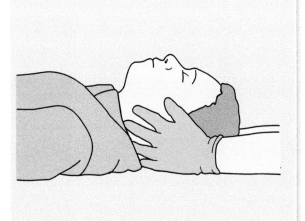

Indications for suctioning

- Noisy breathing
- Excessive secretions that may be visible or audible
- Increased or decreased respirations
- Increased heart rate
- Decreased oxygen saturations
- Prolonged expiratory breath sounds
- Diminished air entry
- Altered chest movements

Children and Young People's Nursing Skills at a Glance, First Edition. Edited by Elizabeth Gormley-Fleming and Deborah Martin.
© 2018 John Wiley & Sons, Ltd. Published 2018 by John Wiley & Sons, Ltd.

Suctioning overview

Normally infants and children have the ability to keep their airways clear of mucus by either coughing, blowing their nose or sneezing. The presence of their gag reflex also prevents harm from secretions in the lower airways. The need to perform oropharyngeal or nasopharyngeal suctioning may arise in the presence of respiratory illness. The child's respiratory system is immature and the altered physiology due to illness may lead to the retention of secretions. If these are not removed, the gaseous exchange may be affected. Suctioning is a traumatic procedure and should only be undertaken when clinically indicated and by experienced practitioners.

Clinical indications

- Noisy breathing.
- Excessive secretions that may be visible or audible.
- Increased or decreased respirations.
- Increased heart rate.
- Decreased oxygen saturations.
- Prolonged expiratory breath sounds.
- Diminished air entry.
- Altered chest movements.

Catheter size and suction pressure

The correct catheter size should be identified and documented. Ideally it should have multiple eyes (two or three) as this will cause less damage than those with a single eye. Multiple eye suction catheters are not required to be rotated during the suctioning procedure. The catheter should always be less than 50% of the airway's internal diameter.

The lowest suction pressure should be used to prevent mucosal trauma. Individual clinical need will also determine the amount of pressure to be used (see Table).

Age	Catheter size	Suction pressure (mmHg)
Neonate	0–5	60–80
Infant: birth–1 year	5–6	80–100
Pre-school	6–8	80–100
School age	8–10	100–120
Adolescent	12 +	120–150

Correct catheter length

- For nasopharyngeal suctioning: pre-measure the catheter from the tip of the child's nose to the suprasternal notch.
- For oropharyngeal suctioning: pre-measure the catheter from the centre of the incisors to the suprasternal notch.
- The length of the suction catheter may be advised by medical staff following certain surgical procedures.

Procedure

- Pre-check all equipment before commencing the procedure.
- Wash and dry your hands and apply personal protective equipment as per local policy.
- Assemble the equipment.
- If possible, sit the child upright. If this is not possible, place the child on their side.
- A second person may be required, one to perform suctioning and one to hold the child safely.
- Remove the oxygen administration devices.
- Pre-oxygenate if required.
- Turn on the suction unit to the required pressure.
- Insert the suction catheter gently, no negative pressure should be applied to the airway at this point.
- Once inserted to the required length, apply negative pressure by occluding the port with your thumb.
- Gently withdraw the catheter. Do not rotate it.
- Assess the effectiveness of the procedure before repeating.
- Repeat the process until the airway is clear. This should be a maximum of three attempts. If this is not sufficient to clear the secretions, then inform medical staff.
- The child should be allowed to recover between each attempt at suctioning.
- Catheters are single use only so must be discarded between each attempt.
- Yankeurs are only used for oral suctioning and must be inserted at the convex angle of the roof of the mouth. They are only used to remove thick secretions/vomitus from the mouth.
- The child should be continually observed and monitored during the procedure. This will include respiratory rate, oxygen saturation levels, heart rate, and colour.
- The colour, amount and viscosity of the secretions should be noted and recorded.
- Clean and dry the nostrils/mouth immediately after the last attempt at suctioning has been completed. The parent/carer may wish to do this.
- Reposition oxygen administration devices and continue to observe the child.
- Flush through suction tubing with sterile water.
- Remove personal protective equipment and discard.
- Wash and dry your hands.
- Document the suction procedure in the child's clinical records.

Complications of suctioning

- Hypoxia.
- Cardiovascular changes.
- Pneumothorax.
- Infection.
- Hypertension/hypotension.
- Trauma to nasal and oral mucosas.
- Raised intracranial pressure.

Key points

- Suctioning should only be performed by competent practitioners.
- The use of an irrigant (0.9% normal saline) may assist with the removal of secretions and should only be used on medical advice and should be prescribed.

32 Tracheostomy care

Tracheostomy position

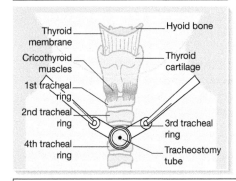

- Thyroid membrane
- Cricothyroid muscles
- 1st tracheal ring
- 2nd tracheal ring
- 4th tracheal ring
- Hyoid bone
- Thyroid cartilage
- 3rd tracheal ring
- Tracheostomy tube

Tracheostomy tube

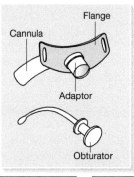

- Cannula
- Flange
- Adaptor
- Obturator

Suction technique

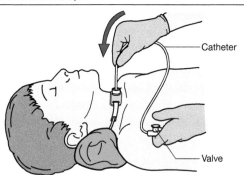

- Catheter
- Valve

Equipment list for tape changes

Tape change equipment:

- Emergency box, oxygen and suction
- Gauze and saline
- 2 lengths of cotton/Velcro ties
- Scissors
- Rolled-up towel
- Blanket for swaddling
- Gloves and apron
- Child's comforter (e.g. dummy)

Tape change procedure

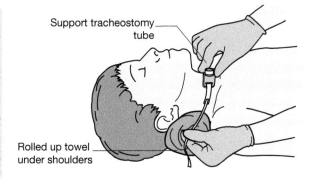

- Support tracheostomy tube
- Rolled up towel under shoulders

Checking tape tension

One finger should slip comfortably between the ties and the child's neck

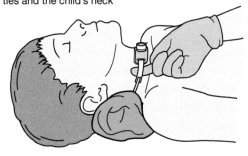
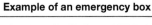

Equipment list for planned tube changes

Tube change equipment:

- Emergency box, oxygen and suction
- A tracheostomy tube same size and one size smaller
- 2 x syringes if child has cuffed tube
- Gauze and saline
- 2 lengths of cotton/Velcro ties
- Scissors
- Rolled-up towel
- Blanket for swaddling
- Gloves and apron
- Child's comforter (e.g. dummy)

Example of an emergency box

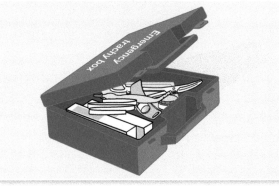

Contents of an emergency box

Emergency tracheostomy box contents:

☑ Same size tracheostomy + smaller size
☑ Tracheostomy tapes
☑ Disconnection wedge
☑ Scissors
☑ Lubricating jelly
☑ Syringes for cuffed tube
☑ Suction catheters

REMEMBER TO ALWAYS KNOW WHERE THE EMERGENCY BOX IS WHEN CARING FOR A CHILD WITH A TRACHEOSTOMY

Children and Young People's Nursing Skills at a Glance, First Edition. Edited by Elizabeth Gormley-Fleming and Deborah Martin.
© 2018 John Wiley & Sons, Ltd. Published 2018 by John Wiley & Sons, Ltd.

Tracheostomy care overview

What is a tracheostomy? A tracheostomy is an opening in the trachea, held open by a tracheostomy tube. Children who require a tracheostomy cannot maintain a patent airway without it, therefore, they need 24-hour care to prevent blockages and other care, including tape/tube changes, care of the stoma and emergency procedures. More and more children with chronic and life-threatening illnesses are surviving each day due to advances in tracheostomy support.

Suctioning

A child with a tracheostomy often finds it hard to clear their own secretions. Suctioning of the tracheostomy tube is an essential part of everyday care to clear secretions from the child's respiratory tract. Airway suctioning can cause serious complications, therefore it should only be carried out when the patency of the airway could be compromised, so you may hear secretions in the tube or see that the child is coughing or having difficulty in breathing.

Suctioning of the tracheostomy tube should be performed as a 'clean technique', wearing gloves. It is essential to remember that children of different ages and sizes will have different sizes of tracheostomy tubes. As a guide, the correct size suction catheter is double the size of their tracheostomy tube, e.g. size 3.5 tracheostomy tube = size 7 fr suction catheter. You also need to know the length of the tracheostomy.

Connect the suction catheter to the suction unit and turn on the suction pressure. Remove the suction catheter without touching the tip of the catheter to keep it sterile. Insert the suction catheter into the tracheostomy tube to the correct depth, indicated by the graduated numbers on the catheter. Once inserted to the correct depth, hold the valve on the suction catheter and slowly withdraw the catheter, while maintaining the vacuum. Once removed, dispose of gloves and the suction catheter appropriately. Suctioning should be a quick and effective procedure of around 5–10 seconds. Ensure you observe the child throughout for any breathing distress or colour change.

Tape changes

Tapes are used to hold the tracheostomy securely in place. Tapes can either be cotton ties or Velcro, different types are used in different hospitals. Tape changes should be carried out daily, with a minimum of two people to carry out the procedure. Infants and some younger children may need to be swaddled, and a rolled-up towel placed under the shoulders to position the airway. It is important to ensure all the equipment is prepared before the procedure begins. Remember to ensure you know where your oxygen and suction are, and have them prepared as they may be needed during the procedure.

One person should be responsible for holding the tracheostomy in place throughout the entire procedure. The other person should be the tape changer. The tape changer should begin by placing clean ties behind the child's neck and cutting the dirty ties off. Then it is important to clean around the tracheostomy site using saline and gauze and dry it thoroughly. While doing this, inspect the condition of the stoma. Sometimes granulation can form where the stoma site is trying to heal, which is often a lump of tissue and this may need treatment. Taking hold of the clean tapes, thread them through and either tie in a bow or Velcro them securely. The 'tension' of the ties must then be checked, by sitting the child up and putting an index finger through the tapes, to make sure they are not too tight or too loose. Readjust them as necessary and then double-bow the cotton tapes and cut the excess so there is 1.25 cm left. The person responsible for holding the tracheostomy MUST NOT let go until told to do so by the tape changer.

Tube changes

Planned tube changes can be done weekly or monthly, depending on the type of tracheostomy tube, and with a minimum of two people. The child should be positioned the same as for the tape change procedure, and all the equipment should be prepared before starting, including oxygen and suction. It is important to know whether the child has a cuffed tube, as this must be deflated prior to removing it. Place clean ties behind the child's neck, and cut the dirty ties, with the assistant holding the tracheostomy secure. The tube changer should have the new tracheostomy to hand, then remove the old one and quickly insert the new one with the obturator in place, in a curved motion. Once inserted, remove the obturator. The assistant should take over holding the tracheostomy in place. The tube changer can then clean the stoma and secure the tracheostomy using the tape change procedure.

Emergency care

All children with a tracheostomy will have an emergency box, which must be kept with them at all times. Most boxes contain a list of what should be included. With an understanding of Basic Life Support (BLS), it can be adapted for a child with a tracheostomy. When checking the airway, check for signs of obstructions like secretions, and suction if necessary. If an obstruction is felt when trying to pass the suction catheter, an emergency tube change may be required. When assessing breathing, if rescue breaths are required, you can deliver them directly to the tracheostomy or by using a bag valve mask (BVM). Another complication in these children can be accidental decannulation, meaning the child could have accidentally removed the tracheostomy or it could have been dislodged. This is when an emergency tube change is required, so use the same size tracheostomy if possible; if not, use the smaller size. Remember to ALWAYS know where the emergency box, oxygen and suction are when caring for a child with a tracheostomy.

Key points
- Dressings should not routinely be used.
- Emergency equipment should always be available and working when caring for a child with a tracheostomy.
- Competency in undertaking this skill is essential when caring for a child with a tracheostomy.

Further reading

Great Ormond Street Hospital (2010) *Living with a Tracheostomy*. Retrieved from: http://www.gosh.nhs.uk/medical-information/procedures-and-treatments/living-with-a-tracheostomy/ (accessed 2 February 2015).

Great Ormond Street Hospital (2012) *Tracheostomy: Care and Management Review*. Retrieved from: http://www.gosh.nhs.uk/health-professionals/clinical-guidelines/tracheostomy-care-and-management-review/ (accessed 2 February 2015).

33 Non-invasive ventilation

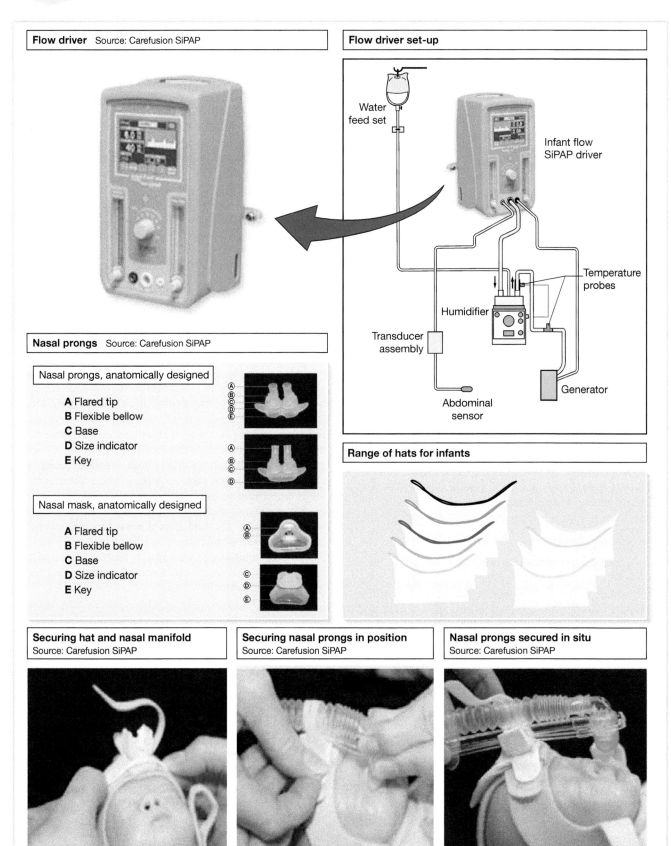

Flow driver   Source: Carefusion SiPAP

Nasal prongs   Source: Carefusion SiPAP

Nasal prongs, anatomically designed

A Flared tip
B Flexible bellow
C Base
D Size indicator
E Key

Nasal mask, anatomically designed

A Flared tip
B Flexible bellow
C Base
D Size indicator
E Key

Flow driver set-up

Water feed set

Infant flow SiPAP driver

Temperature probes

Humidifier

Transducer assembly

Generator

Abdominal sensor

Range of hats for infants

Securing hat and nasal manifold
Source: Carefusion SiPAP

Securing nasal prongs in position
Source: Carefusion SiPAP

Nasal prongs secured in situ
Source: Carefusion SiPAP

Children and Young People's Nursing Skills at a Glance, First Edition. Edited by Elizabeth Gormley-Fleming and Deborah Martin.
© 2018 John Wiley & Sons, Ltd. Published 2018 by John Wiley & Sons, Ltd.

Non-invasive ventilation overview

Non-invasive ventilation (NIV) is used to provide respiratory support in both the acute and chronic (long-term care) settings in infants and children. The term refers to ventilation support that does not involve intubation. Technological advances have resulted in improvements in ventilation strategies that offer a wider range of non-invasive modalities and increased use in children over recent years.

NIV may involve positive airway or negative extrathoracic pressures, although the latter are less commonly used in the United Kingdom. Most NIV involves continuous positive airway pressure (CPAP) or bi-phasic positive airway pressure (BiPAP) delivered by one of a number of fairly simple, portable bedside devices. They are attached to the patient by face or nasal masks or prongs. LCD displays allow adjustment of a few basic settings, such as pressure limits, respiratory rate (for mandatory or back-up ventilation), inspiratory time (Ti) and trigger sensing.

CPAP and BiPAP

CPAP is where a constant positive pressure is applied to the airway of a spontaneously breathing infant or child to maintain adequate end pressure within the alveoli and prevent atelectasis. In current practice, binasal CPAP has superseded the single nasal prong and is most commonly administered non-invasively by a flow driver. The set-up and an example screen can be seen in the Figure. Any mode given via a flow driver should include a humidifier within the circuit to ensure the delivered gases are moistened and warmed to 37 degrees Celsius. The pressure is delivered to the child's airway via two short prongs or a nasal mask. These are attached to the circuit manifold.

Given the relationship between flow and pressure, generally, a flow of 8–10 litres/minute should give a pressure of 4–6 cm/water, provided that there is an adequate seal at the nostrils. Altering the flow will affect the pressure given. For some children, it is necessary to increase the flow to give a higher pressure of 6–7 cm/water (subject to individual assessment by ward medical/nursing team). Oxygen delivery is controlled via a dial.

BiPAP occurs where two pressure levels are set, a background continuous measurement and a higher one, which is delivered at intervals either triggered by the neonate or set as a mandatory 'rate'. Infant Flow SiPAP, for example, provides bi-level nasal CPAP for the spontaneously breathing infant through the delivery of 'pulses' or 'sighs' (brief periods of increased pressure) above a baseline CPAP pressure. These may be timed, or 'triggered' by the infant's own inspiratory efforts.

Flow driver modes

CPAP: This is a mode itself on all ventilators as well as a support strategy in its own right known as nCPAP (nasal CPAP). On the flow driver, it can be given with or without 'apnoea'. If CPAP with apnoea is required, then an abdominal transducer is necessary in order to monitor any apnoeic episode and raise the alarm according to the apnoea time interval, which is set by the user.

BiPAP: The following mode options are available:

• Biphasic-timed: the machine delivers a set baseline pressure using the '*low* pressure' flow metre (set to 8 l/minute on average). The extra pressure-supported 'sighs' are delivered according to a set 'rate' and Ti. The user will set the additional pressure with the '*high* pressure' flow metre which is set at 2 l/minute above the low pressure dial. It is important not to set the 'high pressure' flow too high. The user will also set the number per minute and length of each extra sigh.

• Trigger biphasic: as above but the extra pressure sighs are not timed. These are now triggered by the infant/child initiating a breath.

• Biphasic + apnoea: as for biphasic-timed but there is additional apnoea monitoring and an alarm will sound if the infant/child does not breathe within the apnoea interval.

Application of CPAP and nursing care

The Figure shows how to put the nasal manifold and hat on an infant, as an example. When caring for the infant or child, a balance is necessary between an adequate seal at the nose to maintain pressure and the prevention of nasal trauma.

Procedure

• Ensure the nasal prongs/mask/bonnet are sized correctly according to guidelines.
• Ensure the bonnet-to-nose strapping provides secure fixation but is not too tight.
• Position the neonate and the tubing appropriately so that it is well supported.
• Regularly check for nasal trauma.
• Assess for any discomfort and provide measures to settle and console.
• Continuously monitor vital signs including oxygen monitoring.
• Assess the need for oral/nasal suction only if required.
• Remember mouth care should be given regularly due to potential dryness from gases.
• Continue feeding while on CPAP if applicable – observe for abdominal distention – nasogastric tube should be in situ and left on free drainage if infant/child is not fed OR to be aspirated before each feed and any excess gas removed.
• Once the lungs have improved, provide time off CPAP/BiPAP according to individual care plan and clinical condition. Strategies for weaning pressure and discontinuation of the device are subject to local unit policy.

Key points
• The use of NIV in paediatrics has increased significantly avoiding the necessity for intubation.
• CPAP or BiPAP is a common form of NIV delivery used in infants and children, administered with a flow driver where pressure is set by the application of the gas flow.
• The nursing care of an infant/child on CPAP/BiPAP centres around ensuring optimum respiratory status while protecting them from any undue airway or nasal trauma and discomfort.

Further reading

Hutchings, F. A., Hilliard, T. N. and Davis, P. J. (2014) Heated humidified high-flow nasal cannula therapy in children. *Archives of Disease in Childhood*, **10**, 1–5. DOI:10.1136/archdischild-2014-306590

Petty, J. (2013) Understanding neonatal non-invasive ventilation. *Journal of Neonatal Nursing*, **19**, 10–14.

Samuels, M. and Boit, P. (2007) Non-invasive ventilation in children. *Paediatrics and Child Health*, **17**(5), 167–173.

34 Underwater seal drain

Pleural cavity

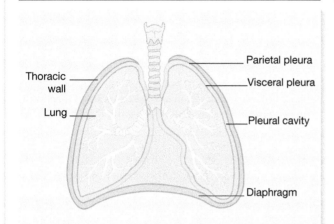

Thoracic wall

Lung

Parietal pleura

Visceral pleura

Pleural cavity

Diaphragm

Simple pneumothorax

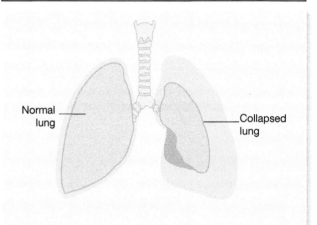

Normal lung

Collapsed lung

Position of chest drain

Insertion of a chest tube: the site is selected in the mid-axillary line in the 5th intercostal space (at the level of the nipple) on the superior aspect of the 6th rib

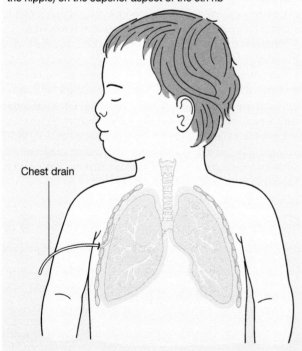

Chest drain

Chest drain and sutures

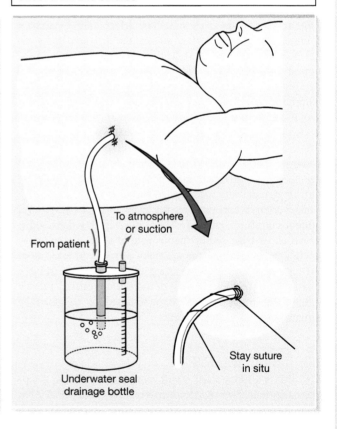

To atmosphere or suction

From patient

Underwater seal drainage bottle

Stay suture in situ

Children and Young People's Nursing Skills at a Glance, First Edition. Edited by Elizabeth Gormley-Fleming and Deborah Martin.
© 2018 John Wiley & Sons, Ltd. Published 2018 by John Wiley & Sons, Ltd.

Underwater seal drain overview

Intra-pleural chest drains are used to treat a child with a collection of fluid or air in the pleural space. This may be due to one of the following clinical conditions:

- simple pneumothorax
- tension pneumothorax
- haemothorax
- pleural effusion
- chylothorax
- emphysema.

Following thoracic or cardiac surgery, a chest drain may also be required.

Intra-pleural chest drains are inserted into the apical pleural space to remove air, or inserted into the basal pleural space to remove fluid. Children requiring a chest drain should be nursed in a high dependency care area. Insertion of the chest drain should be carried out in a tertiary respiratory centre, if their condition permits safe transfer for this procedure.

Once the chest drain has been inserted into the intra-pleural space, it will be attached to drainage tubing that leads into a drainage bottle. The end of this drainage tube will be below the water level. This creates a siphon effect, air or fluid is drawn from the pleural space to the lower level. It is the water in the bottle that creates the underwater seal. This underwater seal prevents air from entering the pleural space. A second tube leads from the drainage bottle. This second tube will either be on low suction or will remain open to the air.

The chest drain is secured to the chest wall by a purse string suture. A sterile waterproof dressing should be applied over the suture.

Position of the chest drain catheter is confirmed by chest X-ray.

Care of the child

- Local policy must be adhered to.
- The drainage tube should be checked hourly and the amount of fluid drained should be recorded. The colour of the fluid should be noted. If there is any increase in the volume of fluid draining, if it becomes blood-stained or if it changes in any way, this will necessitate immediate reporting to medical staff.
- The drainage bottle should be observed at least hourly for a 'swinging' motion to the water. This is due to air leaving the pleural space. This swinging motion decreases as the lung inflates.
- The level of sterile water in the drainage bottle should be recorded on insertion of the chest drain and should not be below the minimum level.
- The amount of fluid (exudate and sterile water) in the drainage bottle should not be more than three-quarters full at any time.

- Aseptic non-touch technique should be employed when changing the bottle.
- The chest tube must be clamped when the bottle is being changed to prevent air entering the pleural cavity via the chest drain.
- Note the amount of sterile water in the bottle when it is connected to the chest drain.
- Where possible, the child should be nursed upright and supported with pillows.
- Vital signs should be recorded as indicated by the child's condition; this should include heart rate, respiratory rate, and oxygen saturation percentage. Temperature should be recorded as a minimum every four hours.
- The work of breathing should be noted, as should the child's colour. Chest movement should be equal. Any shortness of breath or gasping must be reported to medical staff at once.
- Analgesia should be administered as prescribed and its effectiveness noted.
- A keyhole dressing should be in situ over the entry site. The dressing should prevent air from entering the chest cavity. Aseptic non-touch technique should be used for dressing changes and the wound should be kept dry.
- Two clamps must be available at the bedside (flat edges) in case the drainage bottle becomes disconnected.
- If low suction is required, then a low suction unit should be made available.
- Medical staff must prescribe the amount of suction.
- Mobilization is encouraged.
- Physiotherapy may be indicated and care will need to be implemented accordingly.
- A chest X-ray will be required before the removal of the chest drain to ensure the lung has reinflated.
- Removal of the drain will require the suture to be untied. As this is being pulled closed, the drain will be pulled out gently. The co-operation of the child is essential as they will be required to breathe out as the drain is removed. They need to be in a sitting position, leaning forward on a bed table. Analgesia should be administered prior to removal of the drain.
- An occlusive dressing should be applied over the drain site.
- The sutures should be removed as per medical advice. Aseptic non-touch technique should be used.

Key points

- The drainage bottle must never be lifted above the level of the child's chest. There is a risk of water entering the pleural cavity if this occurs.
- A chest drain must never be clamped if the fluid in the underwater seal drain is bubbling or swinging.
- If the chest drain becomes disconnected from the drainage bottle, it must be clamped immediately by placing a clamp on the chest drain just below the entry point.

35 Infant feeding

Healthy and happy infant

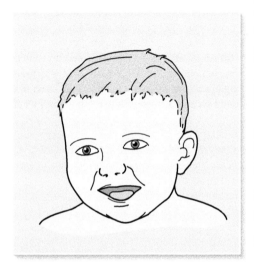

Population of new-borns vs age
Prevalence of any breastfeeding in the United Kingdom in 2010 from birth to 6 months

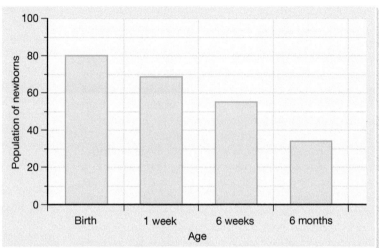

Population of new-borns vs age
Prevalence of exclusive breastfeeding in the United Kingdom in 2010 from birth to 6 months

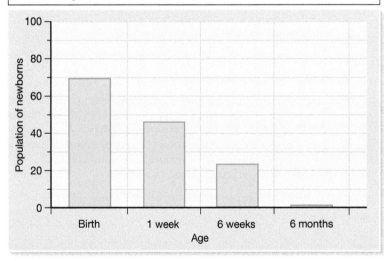

Feeding cues

- Baby waking
- Increased movement as the baby wakes
- Baby moving head around
- Rooting
- Making mouthing movements
- Sucking on fingers
- Crying

Children and Young People's Nursing Skills at a Glance, First Edition. Edited by Elizabeth Gormley-Fleming and Deborah Martin.
© 2018 John Wiley & Sons, Ltd. Published 2018 by John Wiley & Sons, Ltd.

Infant feeding overview

Infant feeding is the means of meeting the nutritional needs of the infant so that they may be healthy and happy. The World Health Organization (2003) recommends exclusive breastfeeding for the first six months of life with the introduction of complementary food after this point, while continuing to breastfeed up till the second birthday or beyond. Other food or drink can be used in the first six months if medically indicated or if there is evidence that the infant is not growing adequately.

In the first six months parents choose either breast (human) milk or artificial formula milk. After six months of age these milks can be used alongside weaning foods. Thus infant feeding incorporates:
• breastfeeding (breastmilk directly from the breast);
• bottle-feeding using artificial formula milk or less commonly breastmilk;
• mixed feeding – breast and artificial formula milk/breastmilk and solids/artificial formula milk and solids.

Choice of feeding method

Parental choice is influenced by a number of physical, emotional and social factors. These include:
• prevailing societal/cultural/family attitudes/practices;
• attitude of partner;
• previous personal experience or having watched close friend or family member feed their baby;
• personal beliefs about their body function and image;
• knowledge of the different methods and their health and social benefits;
• perceived ease or difficulty with breastfeeding/formula feeding;
• media portrayal of infant feeding.
Parents in Britain gain information from a wide variety of sources, such as family and friends, parenting books/magazines, the internet, and health professionals. All of these sources of information can be both accurate and inaccurate. It is recognized that parents face a potential minefield of conflicting information about infant feeding choices and practices.

At the heart of the choice, parents need to be assured that their choice will achieve the following:
• normal pattern of weight gain and growth to achieve regaining birth weight by 2 weeks of age, doubling of birth weight by 6 months and tripling of birth weight by the first birthday;
• normal psychomotor development;
• normal cognitive development;
• happy parent(s) and baby.
While the 'breast is best' message dominates, many parents and professionals perceive artificial formula feeding to be an acceptable, though not best, alternative to breastfeeding.

Commercially manufactured artificial formula milks are the only recommended alternatives to breastmilk. Most formula milk is essentially modified cow's milk. Modification is essential because cow's milk is unsuitable for a baby under one year of age due to higher levels of elements such as sodium. Manufacturers are required to include the type and amount of specific ingredients. For example, the kcal value of the milk must be 60–70 kcal/100 mls – this ensures that any baby will receive sufficient nutrients to maintain their metabolism and grow.

The Infant Feeding surveys undertaken in the United Kingdom every five years have generally indicated that breastfeeding is more likely to be undertaken by women who are older, better educated, married or in a supportive relationship and who are in a higher socio-economic group.

There has been a sustained campaign from the Department of Health to improve the breastfeeding rates. At the last survey in 2010 there was some evidence of this continuing, though when the UK is measured against other countries or the World Health Organization strategy, the picture is not as encouraging. See the Figures for the rates of any breastfeeding from birth to six months with mothers moving from exclusive breastfeeding to the introduction of artificial formula milk on its own or in tandem with some breastfeeding, versus exclusive breastfeeding rates.

Differences between breastmilk and formula milk

While it is accepted that both breastmilk and formula milk will provide nutritional adequacy in relation to protein, fat and carbohydrate composition, there is compelling evidence of the advantages in the 'live' species-specific nature of breastmilk. Breastmilk has immune-enhancing capabilities that extend beyond the colostrum phase. It is nutritionally complete and able to adapt to the changing needs of the baby over time.

Supporting parents

All professionals need to ensure that they are up-to-date with information relating to infant feeding in order to provide parents with evidence-based information and care. They need to respect parental choice and offer support through general information, specific problem-solving in relation to parental care or medical management of conditions as well as providing an environment where parents feel comfortable meeting the nutritional needs of the baby.

Many parents worry about the quantities of milk to feed their baby. Determination of an overall feed can be influenced by the age of the baby/infant, the frequency of feeds, the response to feeding cues, and the baby's satisfaction during and after feeds.

Early recognition of the baby's feeding cues will help parents avoid stressful situations when the baby is upset and crying. This potentially can make feeding a distressing time for all involved and can erode parenting belief.

Key points
• Parental choice is important and support is required as parents often worry if their baby is getting enough nutrition.
• While breastfeeding is natural, it is often difficult for the mother, so additional support may be required.

36 Breastfeeding

Benefits of breastfeeding (UNICEF, 2015)

- Perfectly balanced nutrition for growth and development
- Always at correct temperature
- Always available when mother and baby are together
- Adapts to baby's changing needs
- Reduced risk of some infections
- Reduces risk of infection in baby, e.g., gastroenteritis
- Reduces risk of allergy
- Reduces risk of other conditions in later life, e.g., diabetes mellitus
- Reduces risk of certain cancers in mother, e.g., breast cancer
- Promotes better jaw development and straighter teeth
- Psychologically satisfying, aids bonding

Cross-cradle position with baby in alignment

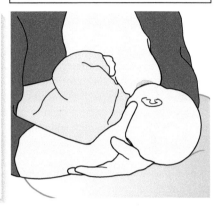

Football position

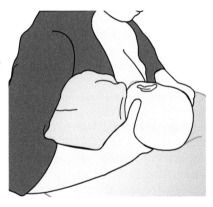

Starting off nose to nipple

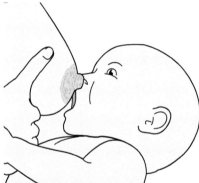

Chin is in good contact with the breast and some areola is visible above the baby's top lip

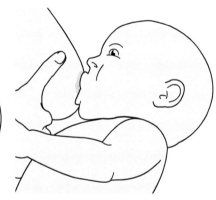

Children and Young People's Nursing Skills at a Glance, First Edition. Edited by Elizabeth Gormley-Fleming and Deborah Martin.
© 2018 John Wiley & Sons, Ltd. Published 2018 by John Wiley & Sons, Ltd.

Breastfeeding overview

Breastfeeding is when the baby is feeding directly at the breast. While it is the biological norm, some mothers do not view breast-feeding as the sociological norm. Breastfeeding is promoted and supported by health professionals in the United Kingdom because of the weight of evidence of the health benefits for baby and mother. Care from health professionals needs to be based on the UNICEF Baby Friendly Initiative Standards (2012). Many maternity units, neonatal units, community services, children's centres and universities training nurses, midwives and health visitors have undergone 'Baby Friendly' accreditation or are working towards it.

Breastmilk

Breastmilk is a live substance made within the mother's breast. It is immediately available to the baby at birth and undergoes changes in the first month of the baby's life. The breastmilk changes are:

- colostrum – present prior to birth and first few days following birth. Present in small amounts, and packed with immunoglobulins. Colostrum is thick and creamy yellow, compared to mature milk, which is thin and bluish in colour.
- transitional milk – by 96 hours to 10–14 days post birth, the colostrum changes to transitional milk.
- mature milk – the type of mother's milk available thereafter until feeding/expressing ceases.

Breastfeeding conveys a range of biological and psychological benefits for the baby and mother (UNICEF, 2015).

Principles to facilitate successful breastfeeding

- Provides skin-to-skin contact between mother and baby.
- It keeps mother and baby close day and night.
- It is baby-led feeding – the mother must watch for feeding cues and respond.
- Mother should be sitting or lying comfortably so that her oxytocin will flow and feeding is sustainable.
- Effective positioning and attachment are required to enable the baby to feed from the breast in an efficient manner and for it to be a pleasant experience for the mother. The baby is positioned in relation to the angle and dangle of the breast to achieve alignment. This will aid a good latch.
- Let the baby finish the first breast before offering the second breast.
- The mother should seek help quickly if experiencing difficulties or is worried about baby not feeding.
- The mother should maintain her milk supply by frequent feeding of baby and by frequent eating and drinking.
- Do not clock-watch when breastfeeding. Keep calm and carry on. Breastmilk production is a supply and demand issue. Feeding at the breast stimulates the release of prolactin from the brain to make the breastmilk and the release of oxytocin to release the milk from the breast. If the baby cannot breastfeed, then the mother needs to maintain her supply by expressing breastmilk using an electric breast pump. Expressing of both breasts simultaneously is more time-efficient.

Feeding/sucking pattern

A healthy baby will initially start feeding at the breast with fast shallow sucks and then change to longer deeper sucks as the milk starts flowing well. The longer, deeper sucking pattern indicates a good 'let-down'. This is when oxytocin has caused the release of the milk from the breast. In the early stages of a feed, there will be short pauses but these will lengthen as the feed progresses and the baby becomes fuller. A sign that the baby may be about to finish the feed is the characteristic fluttering type suck. Many babies can take the majority of milk needed in the first 5–10 minutes of a feed. The feeding frequency will not remain constant. Events such as growth spurts are well recognized to increase feeding frequency while cluster feeding, especially in the evenings, can challenge some mothers. During such episodes it is important to reassure the mother that this is a normal event and to follow cues from the baby. Adjustments of daily life may be needed for maternal peace of mind.

Signs of successful breastfeeding

- A contented baby who wakes to feed and settles between feeds.
- A happy mother.
- Baby having at least six wet nappies and multiple dirty nappies per day (once mature milk is in).
- Baby is growing.

Tips to help mother with feeding

- Try not to separate mother and baby if the baby is admitted to hospital.
- If separated for medical reasons, ensure the mother's milk supply is maintained by pumping.
- If mother requires help with feeding, ensure she has access to a member of staff with additional training to support breastfeeding mothers and babies.
- Different positions to hold baby may help: cross-cradle or football/underarm.
- Is the baby's body close to the mother's body and in alignment with nose and knees pointing in the same direction?
- Is the baby's head able to tilt back and thus help achieve a wide gape?
- Is the baby starting off nose to nipple?
- Once latched, is the angle of the open mouth on the breast the optimal 160 degrees?
- Is the chin tucked into the breast? There should be no space between chin and breast.
- Is the latch comfortable for the mother?
- Is the position sustainable for the mother for the duration of the feed? Mothers generally need to use both arms/hands to support the baby.
- Is the baby actually transferring milk? This is evident by seeing or hearing swallowing, weight gain, wet and dirty nappies.

Breast feeding and HIV

HIV-positive mothers may transmit HIV to their infant during breastfeeding as HIV is found in breastmilk. Emerging evidence now shows that HIV-positive mothers should be encouraged to breastfeed and adhere to their anti-retroviral treatment.

Key points

- Babies with a tongue tie may have difficulties in latching on thus may not be able to feed effectively.
- Breastfeeding is the gold standard of infant feeding.

References

UNICEF (2012) Guide to the Baby Friendly Initiative Standards. Available at: https://www.unicef.org.uk/babyfriendly

UNICEF (2015) *Annual Report*. Available at: https://www.unicef.org/publications/index_92018.html

37 Formula feeding

Mother bottle feeding her baby with formula milk

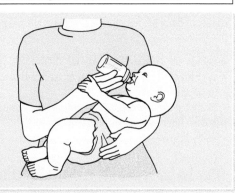

Types of formula milk

- Whey protein-dominant milk
- Casein protein-dominant milk
- First or newborn milk
- Hungrier baby milk
- Follow-on milks
- Pre-term baby milk
- Powdered milk
- Ready-to-feed liquid milk

Formula milk powder with scoop

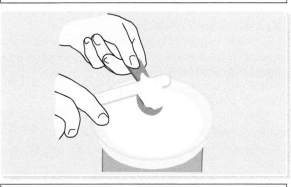

Thorough mixing of water and powder

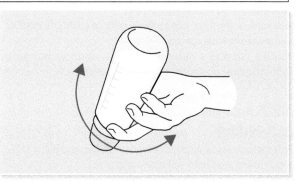

Checking the temperature of the milk

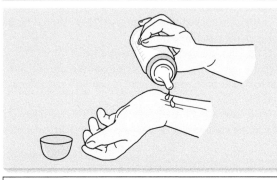

Appropriate feeding technique

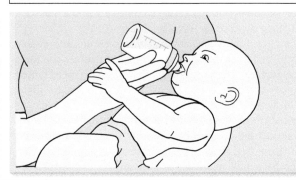

Guide to amount of milk per day

Weight of baby (kg)	Approximate amount of milk per day based on 150 ml/kg/day (ml) (weight x ml/kg/day = amount of daily intake)	Amount per feed based on 6 feeds per day (ml)	Amount per feed based on 8 feeds per day (ml)
3	450 (3 kg x 150 ml)	75	56
4	600 (4 kg x 150 ml)	100	75
5.5	825 (5.5 kg x 150 ml)	137	103

Children and Young People's Nursing Skills at a Glance, First Edition. Edited by Elizabeth Gormley-Fleming and Deborah Martin.
© 2018 John Wiley & Sons, Ltd. Published 2018 by John Wiley & Sons, Ltd.

Formula feeding overview

Formula feeding is generally viewed as the delivery of artificial formula milk via a feeding bottle and teat to the baby.

In helping parents to safely feed their baby using formula milk, the following factors are important:
• information regarding the type of formula milk to use that is appropriate for their baby's age/stage of development and any medical issues known;
• how to sterilize all feeding equipment;
• information on how to prepare formula feeds if using a powder or liquid concentrate preparation;
• techniques to physically feed the baby in a safe manner that also promotes parent–baby relationship;
• how much to feed their baby.

Types of formula milk

There are numerous brands of artificial formula milk available to parents in the United Kingdom. The milks can be classified in a number of ways. Whey protein-dominant milks are thought to be closer to the make-up of breast milk and thus are easier to digest. Thus they are advised for newborns. First milks are able to be used from birth to the first birthday when cow's milk can be introduced. Casein protein-dominant milks are marketed for hungry babies as it is claimed that the higher proportion of casein takes longer to digest and the baby stays fuller longer and sleeps longer. There is no evidence that it is superior to first milks. Follow-on milks are marketed for use from six months of age.

Generally parents will use a powdered form that needs reconstituting before it can be fed to the baby. Such tins/packets of formula powder will come with manufacturer's instructions for reconstitution and a plastic scoop for measuring the powder.

Sterilizing equipment

Sterilizing all feeding equipment is important as the baby's immune system is still immature. The major threat to a baby is from gastroenteritis. Fungal infections may also possibly be transmitted via feeding equipment. The steps in achieving a satisfactory level of sterilization are as follows:
• Discard leftover feed.
• Rinse bottle and teat thoroughly.
• Wash in hot soapy water using a bottle brush to clean inside the bottle, around the neck of the bottle and use a teat brush (often on the other end of the bottle brush) to clean both the outside and the inside of the teat.
• Rinse all the cleaned equipment to remove soap.
• Use the chosen method of sterilization.
Sterilization may be achieved by one of the following methods:
• chemical sterilization using cold tap water and a sterilizing liquid or tablet;
• steam sterilizing using a microwave or an electric steam sterilizer;
• boiling in a saucepan for at least 10 minutes.

Preparation of feeds

Current advice is to make up each feed as the baby needs it. Key points to remember are:
• Boil the kettle with the required amount of water and leave it to cool for up to 30 minutes before pouring the required amount into bottle.
• Wash your hands and clean the surface to be used to prepare the feed.
• Measure out the required number of scoops of powder, levelling each scoop with the leveller and avoiding compression in the scoop. Generally use one scoop of powder for each fluid ounce of water.
• Ensure that when placing the teat and screw ring on the top of the bottle that the teat does not touch anything.
• Shake well to mix the powder and water thoroughly.

Feeding the baby

There are key safety issues involved in feeding the baby. After preparation of the feed, the temperature of the milk should be checked. Using the inside of your wrist is ideal because the skin in that area is sensitive to temperature. The milk should feel warm rather than hot on your inside wrist. If the milk is too hot, cool the bottle under cold running water and recheck it before feeding starts. The milk should never be made up hours in advance and stored in the fridge due to the risks of bacterial contamination of the powder by organisms such as Enterobacter sakazakii and Salmonella. Equally there is danger from warming chilled feeds using a microwave due to the risks of hotspots that may not be identified when the temperature of the milk is checked on the inside of the wrist.

Babies being fed artificial formula milk should be fed using a demand feeding approach. In this way the baby is able to vary the frequency of feeds and the amount taken at each feed. Observing for early feeding cues is important in order to have time to prepare a fresh feed.

The baby should be clean, dry, and warm and calm prior to the feed. It is an important time of communication between parent and baby and both mother and baby should enjoy the relaxed time. Prop feeding should never be undertaken as there is a risk of choking.

The bottle teat should be placed at the baby's lips and when the mouth opens, slide the teat into the mouth so that it sits on the upper side of the tongue. It is important to avoid pushing the teat too far back into the baby's mouth or the gag reflex will be stimulated. The bottle can then be tipped upwards until the flanged area of the teat fills with milk – this avoids excessive ingestion of air. The flow of the teat should be sufficient to provide well-formed drops of milk rather than an overwhelming rush of milk. The baby should be allowed to pace the feed with pauses between sucking bursts and will indicate when they have had sufficient. Burping, or winding, can be undertaken at the end of the feed or periodically during a feed.

How much to feed the baby

This will depend on age, appetite, feeding frequency and the individual preference of the baby. From 1 week to 6 months, a baby will need 150–200 mls/kg/day to meet nutritional needs.

Key points
• Feed requirements are dependent on the weight of the baby.
• Safety is paramount in all aspects of formula feeding: from preparation of the formula to positioning of the baby for feeding.

38 Insertion of nasogastric and nasojejunal tubes

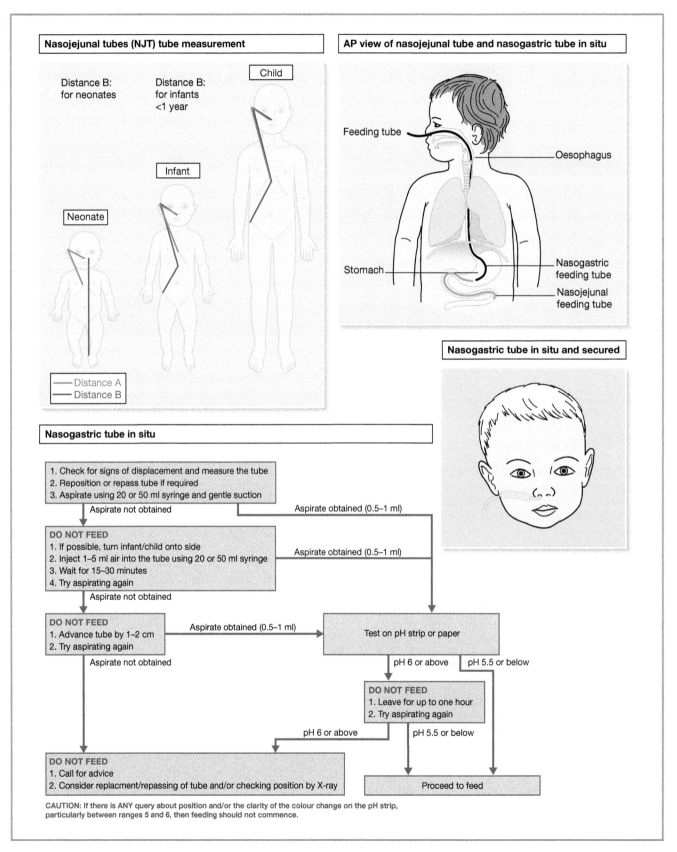

Nasojejunal tubes (NJT) tube measurement

Distance B: for neonates

Distance B: for infants <1 year

Child

Infant

Neonate

— Distance A
— Distance B

AP view of nasojejunal tube and nasogastric tube in situ

Feeding tube

Oesophagus

Stomach

Nasogastric feeding tube

Nasojejunal feeding tube

Nasogastric tube in situ and secured

Nasogastric tube in situ

1. Check for signs of displacement and measure the tube
2. Reposition or repass tube if required
3. Aspirate using 20 or 50 ml syringe and gentle suction

Aspirate not obtained

Aspirate obtained (0.5–1 ml)

DO NOT FEED
1. If possible, turn infant/child onto side
2. Inject 1–5 ml air into the tube using 20 or 50 ml syringe
3. Wait for 15–30 minutes
4. Try aspirating again

Aspirate obtained (0.5–1 ml)

Aspirate not obtained

DO NOT FEED
1. Advance tube by 1–2 cm
2. Try aspirating again

Aspirate obtained (0.5–1 ml)

Test on pH strip or paper

Aspirate not obtained

pH 6 or above

pH 5.5 or below

DO NOT FEED
1. Leave for up to one hour
2. Try aspirating again

pH 6 or above

pH 5.5 or below

DO NOT FEED
1. Call for advice
2. Consider replacment/repassing of tube and/or checking position by X-ray

Proceed to feed

CAUTION: If there is ANY query about position and/or the clarity of the colour change on the pH strip, particularly between ranges 5 and 6, then feeding should not commence.

Children and Young People's Nursing Skills at a Glance, First Edition. Edited by Elizabeth Gormley-Fleming and Deborah Martin.
© 2018 John Wiley & Sons, Ltd. Published 2018 by John Wiley & Sons, Ltd.

Insertion of nasogastric and nasojejunal tubes overview

A nasogastric tube (NGT) is a long tube that is passed through the nasal passage, the oesophagus and into the stomach. It has two main uses; feeding and emptying of stomach contents.

NGTs come in a variety of sizes of diameters. Some tubes will also have a guidewire to help aid insertion. The size used will depend on the size of the child's nostril and the measured landmarks for insertion.

NGTs are intended for short-term use. If the child requires a longer-term method of enteral feeding the child will be assessed for a gastrostomy.

It is vital that staff are trained and competent in passing NGTs and checking the correct positioning. It is important to communicate the purpose of NGT with the child and carer and to obtain consent.

Equipment

Gloves and apron, NGT (of appropriate size), sterile water, tapes, 20 ml enteral syringe, pH testing paper, a dummy, bottle, or glass of water and a straw (dependent on age).

Insertion

Prior to insertion the tip of the NGT should be placed on the tip of the child's nose and then measured to the tragus of the ear and down to the xiphisternum (where the ribs meet in the centre of the chest). A note should be taken of the number on the tube.

The child, depending on age, can be held by a parent/carer, ideally in an upright position but young babies may be swaddled and laid flat. The tip of the tube may have a light coating of sterile water applied to act as a lubricant to ease insertion through the nasal passage and should be passed through the larger of the nostrils along the floor of the nasal passage. The tube should be pushed slowly and not forced, past the back of the nostril. It may be useful at this point to try and encourage the child to suck a dummy or drink from a cup/bottle to help aid the NGT into the oesophagus and down into the stomach. This is then taped to the child's face/cheek, once the required measurement on the NGT reaches the nostril.

To check for correct positioning, the 20 ml syringe should be connected to the end of the NGT and an aspirate obtained. This should be tested with pH paper. Correct positioning will give a reading of between pH 1–5.5 and is a reliable indicator in determining whether the tube is in or outside the stomach. However, X-ray remains the gold standard.

The tube should be checked at the following times:
• following the initial placement;
• before administering each feed or any medication;
• at least once a day if the patient is receiving a continuous feed;
• following an episode of vomiting/coughing;
• if there is any evidence that the tube has been displaced.
The correct procedure shows a sufficient aspirate of between 0.5–1 ml and this should be documented in the patient's notes.

Orogastric tubes

Sometimes it is not appropriate to use the nostril for the insertion of an NGT, e.g. if a child is receiving CPAP, has a narrowing of a nasal passage (coanal atresia) or if there is any suspicion of a basal skill fracture. In this case the tube can be inserted via the child's mouth in the same way as it would be nasally, with the exception that it is measured from the mouth to the tragus and xiphisternum.

Nasojejunal tubes (NJT)

Jejunal tube feeding is used to feed directly into the small bowel. It is indicated if a child has delayed gastric emptying, persistent vomiting, severe gastro-oesophageal reflux or in the presence or an absence of the gag reflex.

Similar to placing an NGT, it is important to inform the child family of the need for the NJT, how it will be placed and to gain consent.

Equipment

The equipment required is the same as that for an NGT but a nasojejunal tube is used.

Procedure

The NGT tube should be measured prior to insertion. This should be done by taking two measurements. The first measurement (distance A) is taken the same way that you would measure for an NGT. The second measurement (distance B) is measured according to age.

Insertion

The child should be laid on their right side with a head elevation of 15–30 degrees if possible. Pass the tube as if inserting an NGT to distance A and secure. An aspirate should be obtained of a reading of <5.5 pH. Once placement has been confirmed, a small flush of water (2 ml in child, 0.5 ml in a neonate) should be given to encourage peristalsis and then slowly the tube should be advanced by:
• 1 cm every 15–30 mins for neonates;
• 2–4 cm every 5–10 mins for an infant and small child;
• 4–6 cm every 5–10 mins for a bigger child
Flush with water prior to advancing each time until distance B is reached. Following insertion of the tube, it should be checked for placement via either a fluoroscopy or an extended chest X-ray. This should occur approximately one hour post insertion to allow time for peristalsis to move the tube through the pylorus.

A clinician experienced in the assessment of NJT placement should interpret the X-ray and confirm placement.

The procedure and measurements should be documented in the patient's notes.

The NJT should not be checked by obtaining an aspirate as this can cause the tube to recoil. A visual check of the tube is necessary, checking the marked measurement at the nostril and ensuring there has been no displacement of the tube every time the tube is used and/or at least daily.

NJT cannot be used for bolus feeding due to the jejunum having no capacity and this may cause vomiting, diarrhoea and abdominal pain. Feeds should therefore be administered continuously via a feeding pump. Care should also be taken to ensure that feeds are prepared and given in a sterile manner as the NJT bypasses the natural microbiological defences of the stomach.

Key points
• The tube position must be confirmed before it is used either by pH testing or X-ray confirmation.
• The infant/child should be observed for signs of vagal stimulation during insertion and, if evident. the procedure must be stopped until the infant/child has been assessed and recovered.

Further reading

National Patient Safety Agency (NPSA) (2005) *Reducing Harm Caused by the Misplacement of Nasogastric Feeding Tubes: How to Confirm the Correct Position of Nasogastric Feeding Tubes in Infants, Children and Adults*. London. NHS.

39 Nasogastric tube feeding

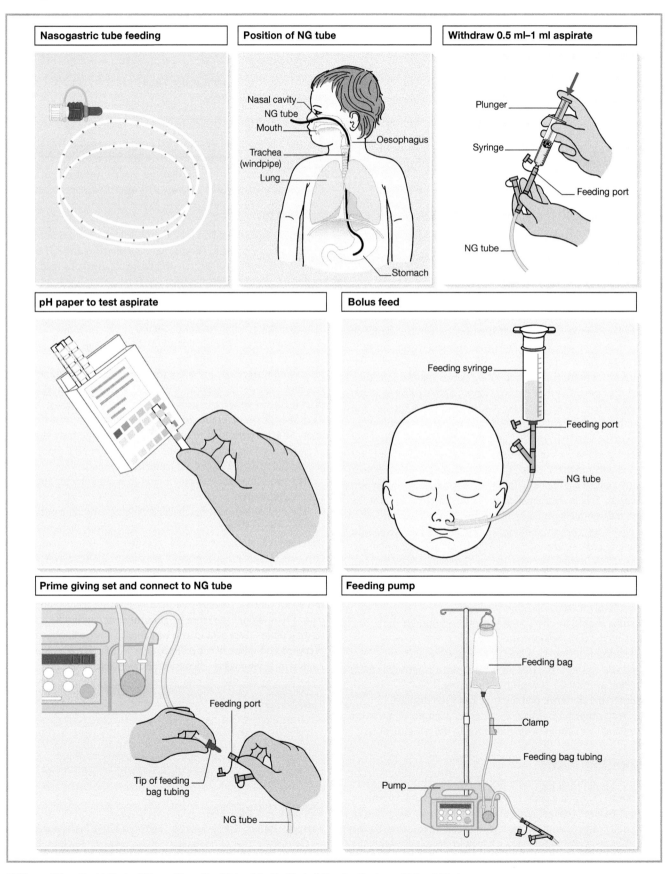

Nasogastric tube feeding

Position of NG tube

Nasal cavity
NG tube
Mouth
Trachea (windpipe)
Lung
Oesophagus
Stomach

Withdraw 0.5 ml–1 ml aspirate

Plunger
Syringe
Feeding port
NG tube

pH paper to test aspirate

Bolus feed

Feeding syringe
Feeding port
NG tube

Prime giving set and connect to NG tube

Feeding port
Tip of feeding bag tubing
NG tube

Feeding pump

Feeding bag
Clamp
Feeding bag tubing
Pump

Children and Young People's Nursing Skills at a Glance, First Edition. Edited by Elizabeth Gormley-Fleming and Deborah Martin.
© 2018 John Wiley & Sons, Ltd. Published 2018 by John Wiley & Sons, Ltd.

Nasogastric tube feeding overview

A nasogastric (NG) tube is a polyurethane or silicone tube that is inserted into the stomach via the nasal passage. Orogastric tubes may also be used particularly if the nasal passages are compromised or being used to administer oxygen, e.g. CPAP. The two main reasons for using a NG tube are:

1 to supply nutrition;
2 to empty the gastrointestinal tract.

Infants and children can be fed via a nasogastric tube either totally or partially. The feeds can be given via gravity or via a pump on an intermittent or on a continuous basis.

Equipment

Plastic apron and gloves
Clear work surface, i.e. tray
20–50 ml syringes
Sterile water
pH indicator paper and comparison chart (CE marked paper)
Feed as prescribed
Pump – continuous feed
Giving set – bolus, intermittent feed

Procedure

Before commencing a feed, the position of the tube must be confirmed. This will be done by aspirating the gastric secretions. Parental consent should be obtained and also the consent of the child should be obtained. Ensure the child is in a comfortable position, ideally sitting on their parent's knee if possible. If in a bed or cot, then tilt the head of the bed/cot to a 45° angle so as to prevent aspiration.

Local policy should be followed:

• Wash hands and put on apron and gloves.
• Connect the 20 ml syringe to the port of the NG tube and aspirate 0.5–1 ml of gastric contents.
• Drop onto the pH paper and match the colour to the comparison chart. The pH should be below 5.5 for infants (term) and children.

Bolus feed

Remove the giving set and using the aseptic non-touch technique attach the 50 ml syringe to the top of the giving set. Prime the line with the feed and the clamp. Attach the giving set to the NG tube. Unclamp the giving set and administer the feed.

If you are not using a giving set, then attach the 50 ml syringe to the top of the NG tube. Kink the NG tube and pour the feed into the syringe. Release the NG tube and allow the feed to flow into the child's stomach. The rate of administration of the NG feed should take roughly the same length of time that it would take the infant/child to feed. This will depend on the viscosity of the feed, the size of the NG tube and the height of the syringe. Thickening agents added to the feed will lead to a slower rate of flow.

Continuous feeding

Using the aseptic non-touch technique, remove the feeding set from its packaging. Close the clamp. Attach to the feeding reservoir and the prime chamber. Unclamp and allow the feed to flow through the line to prime it. Label the line with the date and time.

Insert the feeding set into administration pump. Connect the feeding set to the nasogastric tube. Set the pump to the prescribed rate and commence the feed. Continue to observe the child closely initially and in accordance with the local policy. Any increase in the work of breathing or other changes to the child's condition should be reported and the feed stopped at once.

Flushing out the NG tube

Once the feed is finished, the tube should be flushed out as per the local policy, this is usually with sterile water and the volume will depend on the age of the child.

All equipment should be discarded and hands should be washed.

The amount of feed given, the type of feed, the amount of flush used and how the child tolerated the feed should be documented in the child's notes.

Key points

• The position of the NG tube must be checked prior to its use on each occasion.
• If there is any doubt about its position, it should not be used until it has been confirmed to be in the stomach. This may require re-insertion or X-ray confirmation.
• Mouth care should be initiated for the child who is unable to feed orally.
• Local policy must be adhered to.
• Neonates have different physiology so specific guidance must be adhered to.

Further reading

National Patient Safety Agency (NPSA) (2005) Reducing the harm caused by misplaced naso and orogastric feeding tubes in babies under the care of neonatal units. Patient Safety Alert NPSA/2005/9. London: NPSA.

National Patient Safety Agency (NPSA) (2011) Reducing the harm caused by misplaced nasogastric feeding tubes in adults, children and infants. Patient Safety Alert NPSA/2011/PSA002. London: NPSA.

40 Gastrostomy feeding

Gastrostomy tube

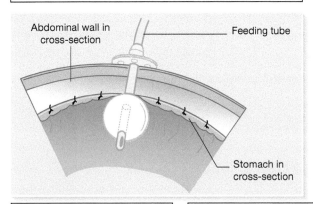

Abdominal wall in cross-section

Feeding tube

Stomach in cross-section

Partial and Full Buried Bumper Syndrome

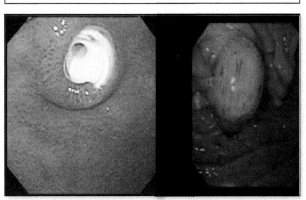

Stoma sites should be monitored daily for the following signs

- Inflammation
- Erythema
- Heat
- Swelling
- Exudate
- Over-granulation
- Leakage and excoriation
- Pressure damage
- Discomfort and pain

Balloon-retained devices

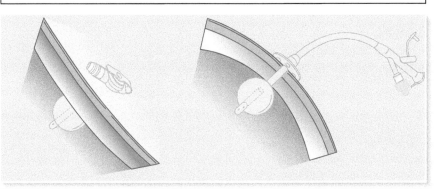

Granulation tissue

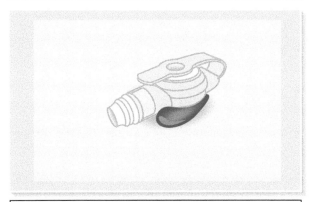

Gastrostomy tube secured with a dressing and securement device

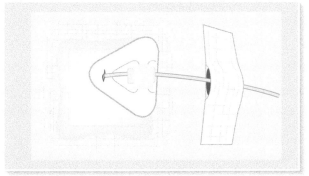

Excoriated site due to leakage of gastric contents

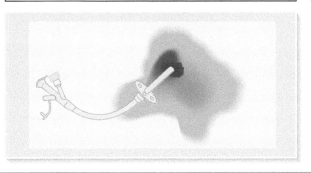

Stoma site infection

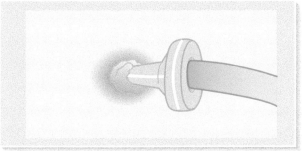

Children and Young People's Nursing Skills at a Glance, First Edition. Edited by Elizabeth Gormley-Fleming and Deborah Martin.
© 2018 John Wiley & Sons, Ltd. Published 2018 by John Wiley & Sons, Ltd.

Gastrostomy feeding overview

A gastrostomy is a surgically formed artificial opening into the stomach known as a stoma. They are commonly surgically inserted endoscopically through the abdominal wall, and held in place by an internal balloon or bumper and external fixator. Gastrostomy feeding is a successful method of enteral feeding providing daily nutritional requirements in specialist liquid form directly into a patient's stomach via a flexible tube.

It is a method that should be considered in patients likely to need long-term (4 weeks or more) enteral tube feeding. The decision concerning the placement of a gastrostomy is usually dependent on the estimated length of therapy, and the needs of the parent and caregivers.

The tubes come in a variety of types and are referred to according to the type inserted. The commonest types are percutaneous endoscopic gastrostomy (PEG) tubes and low-profile gastrostomy tubes, e.g. Mic-key button™.

When it is decided that a patient requires gastrostomy feeding, the type of feed they receive will differ according to their individual requirements in consultation with a dietician and consultant.

There are two main methods of feeding via a gastrostomy as detailed below:
* *Bolus feeding*: A volume of liquid feed given usually via a gravity set over a short duration, e.g. 15–20 minutes.
* *Continuous feed*: This is a feed given via an electronic feeding pump, which allows clinicians and home caregivers to deliver set amounts of enteral formula in a consistent manner, over a desired duration of time.

Preparation and equipment

Before administration of feed, preparation is paramount, therefore simple steps should be adopted as detailed below:
* Collect the appropriate equipment, e.g. syringes (20–50 ml), gravity feeding set, pump, pump feeding set, gloves, apron, water for flush.
* Make feed or use appropriate pre-made feed.
* Check the expiry date of the feed.
* Gain informed consent from patient or parent prior to administration of feed.

Procedure for bolus feed

* Wash hands in accordance with local hand hygiene policy.
* Put on gloves and apron.
* Ensure the patient is sitting up or elevated as much as their condition dictates, to help prevent vomiting and aspiration during the feed and for a period of time after the feed is completed.
* Flush the gastrostomy with approx. 10 ml of water to confirm the patency of the tube.
* Open the gravity feeding pack, which should consist of:
  * 60 ml open-ended syringe;
  * extension tubing with a roller clamp system;
  * Luer lock connector end, with purple and clear capped end.
* Taking the tubing, ensure the clamp is rolled in a downward position, connect the bladder tip syringe on to the open end of the tubing.
* Take your feed, pour enough feed into the syringe to cover the stretch of the tubing and a little bit more approx. 15 ml.
* Over the sink, roll the clamp slowly into the upward position and gradually prime the tubing till it reaches the Luer lock end.
* Ensure the clamp is in the downward position.

* Attach the Luer lock end to the appropriate enteral feeding port on the gastrostomy.
* Unclamp, then clamp on the gastrostomy tube.
* Hold the syringe with the feed up and gradually release the clamp until fully open. Reducing the height of where the syringe is held will slow down the speed at which the feed is administered.
* Once the volume of feed is delivered, clamp down on the administration tube before the milk reaches the end, and close the clamp on the gastrostomy extension.
* Remove the giving set and flush the gastrostomy using an oral 20 ml syringe filled with a minimum of 10 ml water (sterile or cooled boiled water for children under the age of one).

Procedure for a pump feed

* Collect all the relevant equipment required for the feed as per the bolus feed, including the feeding pump.
* Wash hands in accordance with local hand hygiene policy.
* Put on gloves and apron.
* Ensure the patient is sitting up or elevated as much as their condition dictates, to help prevent vomiting and aspiration during the feed and for a period of time after the feed is completed.
* Flush the gastrostomy with approx. 10 ml of water to confirm the patency of the tube.
* Take the feed and the feeding set.
* The tubing extension will have a purple screw top, with a sharp pointed skewer, a length of tubing with a plastic chamber below the cap and a purple kite-shaped junction half-way down the tubing with a squeezable priming attachment.
* The feed will either need to be decanted into a plastic bottle that will be provided with the extension or will come in a pre-made bottle with a foil seal.
* Connect the tubing onto the feed.
* Half-fill the plastic chamber with milk by squeezing the sides.
* Hold the milk up in the air, and using the squeezable primer, push until the tubing is fully purged of air and full of milk, ensuring to stop just after the junction.
* In accordance with the manufacturer's guidelines for the pump, attach the bottle/bag to the pump and set the rate and the total volume of feed to be delivered. Ensure the pump is set to hold.
* Attach the Luer lock end to the appropriate enteral feeding port on the gastrostomy.
* Unclamp, then clamp on the gastrostomy tube.
* Ensure the clamp is released on the gastrostomy extension if relevant, and turn the pump dial to run.
* Once the volume of feed is delivered, close the clamp on the gastrostomy extension and detach from the pump.
* Remove the giving set and flush the gastrostomy using an oral 20 ml syringe filled with a minimum of 10 ml water (sterile or cooled boiled water for children under the age of one).

Key points
* You do not need to test an aspirate of a gastrostomy as it is directly inserted into the stomach.
* Flushing is a vital component of feeding via a gastrostomy. It helps maintain the patency of the tube, preventing the common problem of tube blockage.
* The enteral syringe used should not be less than a 20 ml syringe. This is important to reduce the pressure exerted, minimizing the risk of damage to the stomach wall.
* Complaints of pain or leakage of feed from the stoma site, could indicate there is a problem with the patient's gastrostomy. Stop the feed immediately and seek help.

41 Urine collection

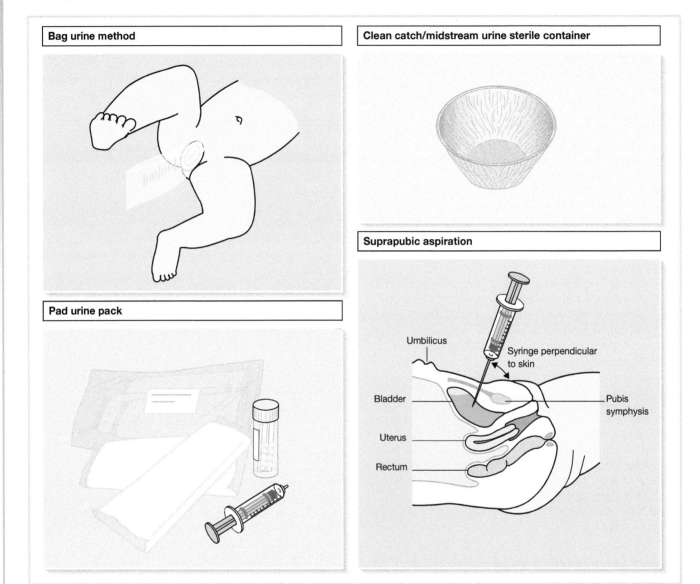

Bag urine method

Clean catch/midstream urine sterile container

Pad urine pack

Suprapubic aspiration

Umbilicus

Syringe perpendicular to skin

Bladder

Pubis symphysis

Uterus

Rectum

Urine collection overview

Collecting a urine sample from a child is a fundamental skill for children's nurse, however, collecting a suitable specimen can be challenging. The urine collected should, whenever possible, be a midstream or clean catch sample to ensure there is no contamination from external contact. Children's nurses need skills of communication, patience and clear explanations to support children of all ages and their parents to cooperate with the task in hand.

Urine is collected for many reasons:

- as part of a septic screen;
- for urinalysis;
- for culture in the laboratory.

General principles

- Following clear explanations, verbal consent should be obtained from the child and the parent.

- A risk assessment should be considered to ensure contamination or cross-infection does not occur.
- Privacy and dignity should be considered and maintained throughout the procedure.
- Consider what assistance may be required and from whom, the children's nurse or parent, ensure the parent is well informed of the procedure especially in relation to cross-contamination.
- A pain assessment may be required prior to a suprapubic specimen being obtained.
- Hands should be washed in line with national guidelines and personal protection equipment, disposable aprons and gloves must be worn.
- Local policies should be adhered to.
- Specimens for the laboratory should be transported safely, without risk to carrier or the receiver.
- Specimen containers must be secured properly to prevent risk of spillage and double-sided polythene bags should be used.

Children and Young People's Nursing Skills at a Glance, First Edition. Edited by Elizabeth Gormley-Fleming and Deborah Martin.
© 2018 John Wiley & Sons, Ltd. Published 2018 by John Wiley & Sons, Ltd.

- Specimens need to be clearly labelled with the child's name, hospital number and date of birth, along with date and time of collection, type of specimen.
- Specimens to be sent to the laboratory need to be accompanied by the appropriate and accurately completed form.
- Document, with date and time, in medical notes that a specimen of urine has been collected, ward tested (with result) and sent to the laboratory.

Shared methodology

- Ensure the child and their parents understand the reasons for collecting the specimen.
- Ensure all involved understand how the urine is going to be collected.
- The genitalia in all cases should be washed and dried carefully, no creams or powder to be applied.
- The children's nurse and/or the parent must also wash their hands.

Methods of collection

Bag urine

An adhesive bag is attached to the baby's genitalia. The accuracy of this method is debatable with many false positive results obtained due to contamination.

Procedure

- Apply the adhesive bag securely to the baby's genitalia:
  - Girl – apply first to the perineum and then over the vulva.
  - Boy – insert the penis into the bag and stick down firmly.
- Ensure there are no creases to prevent the skin becoming sore.
- Check the bag regularly and remove as soon as the baby has passed urine.
- If the urine is contaminated with faeces, the process will need to be repeated.
- Transfer urine to sterile specimen pot.
- Wash and apply cream to the baby before reapplying a nappy.

Clean catch/midstream urine

A clean catch or midstream urine sample is the recommended method for urine collection. The method used will depend on the age of the child.

Toilet-trained/older child

- Ensure they have a suitable sterile container to collect the urine, and check that the child understands the importance of not contaminating the container.
- The child should pass a small amount of urine into the toilet; this eliminates bacteria from the per-urethral area.
- The sterile container is used to catch the middle stream of urine.
- The child continues to empty his/her bladder in the usual way.

The younger child

- As above, except the parent/nurse removes the nappy from the child and waits to 'catch' the urine in the sterile container.
- Giving the child drinks at this time may hasten the process.

Pad urine

A sterile pad is placed in the baby's nappy.

Procedure

- Place the sterile pad inside the nappy, taking care not to contaminate the pad by touching it.

- The nappy should be inside out to allow the pad to absorb all the urine.
- Check the pad regularly and remove when the pad is wet.
- Replace pad after 30 minutes if the child has not passed urine to prevent contamination from skin flora.
- Using the sterile syringe supplied in the pack, withdraw the urine from the pad and place in the sterile urine container. This may have to be repeated several times until enough urine is extracted for testing.
- If the pad is contaminated with faeces, it needs to be discarded and the process started again.

Suprapubic aspiration (SPA)

SPA may be described as the gold standard for collecting a sterile urine sample from a child, however, it is painful, invasive and not without risk and is therefore not commonly performed in general paediatrics. When it is not possible or practical to collect urine by non-invasive methods, catheter samples or suprapubic aspiration (SPA) should be used. SPA is a medical procedure although the children's nurse will be required to reassure and provide explanations to the family and to hold the baby in the supine position with legs extended. It is recommended that a scanner is used to ascertain if the baby's bladder contains urine. The skin should be cleaned using an alcohol swab and allowed to dry. A 23-G needle with syringe attached is inserted through the abdominal wall into the child's bladder and the urine withdrawn. A small plaster is applied after the procedure.

Points to note

- Analgesia may be required prior to the procedure.
- The parents should be warned that haematuria (blood in the urine) may occur after the event.
- Localised bleeding may occur.

Throughout the preparation and during the procedure, someone should be available to catch some urine as the child may pass urine at any time during the process.

Catheter specimen of urine (CSU)

If a child already has a urinary catheter, a sample of urine can be obtained from the sampling port on the catheter tubing, this may require a needle and syringe or may be a needleless port.

Procedure

- Use universal precautions of wearing an apron and gloves.
- If available, clamp the urinary drainage tube below the sampling port to allow the urine to collect in the tube.
- Clean the sampling port using an alcohol swab and allow to dry.
- Either insert a needle at 45° angle, to prevent needle piercing the tubing wall, or use the needleless port.
- Withdraw urine into the syringe, remove the needle and swab the area with a clean alcohol swab and leave to dry.
- Unclamp the drainage tube.
- Put urine into sterile collecting pot and safely discard needle and syringe.
- Do not collect samples from the drainage bag as these are likely to be stale and contaminated.

Key points

- While urine collection is a common procedure in children's nursing, it is important that children's nurses consider their patient when deciding on the most suitable collection method.
- Following the correct guidelines ensures that contamination is kept to a minimum, allowing accurate urinalysis or laboratory results.

42 Catheter insertion

Insertion of a catheter

Insertion of a urinary catheter is an invasive, unpleasant procedure for a child and family. Care must be taken to minimize trauma and distress. Children's nurses carrying out this procedure need to be aware of their own level of competence, have an understanding of their accountability and responsibility in relation to national legislation, national guidelines and local policies.

Fully explain the procedure to the child and/or family, ensuring they understand the reason for needing the catheter. Allow time for questions.

Gain verbal consent from the child and family (where appropriate).

Consider the need for restraining the child and/or therapeutic holding, gain consent for this and ensure the child's rights and safety are maintained.

Consider the age and development of the child, think whether play preparation would be beneficial.

Maintain dignity and privacy throughout.

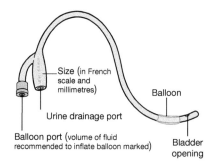

Prepare all equipment giving careful consideration to the most appropriate catheter to use.

Ensure the child has no allergies to latex, the cleansing solutions or any adhesive tape to be used.

Urinary catheterization is associated with increased risk of acquiring a hospital infection, therefore, it is important to maintain sterility throughout the procedure.

Variations for a girl

It's important to understand the anatomy of the female to avoid inserting the catheter into the vagina. If this does occur, leave the catheter in place to prevent it happening again and insert a new catheter into the urethral opening.

Ask the girl to lie supine with knees bent and flexed outwards.

Using the non-dominant hand, hold the labia open with sterile gauze.

Clean, using a sterile solution, first, the outer labia, then the inner labia, and finally the vulvar groove.

Use a new piece of gauze each time and wipe front to back.

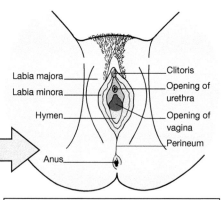

Cleaning solution

It is widely acceptable for sterile normal saline to be used to clean the urethral areas, however, children's nurses need to be aware of local policies in relation to using saline over an antiseptic solution.

Variations for a boy

Knowledge of anatomy is important, the foreskin or prepuce will not retract in boys under five years and forcing it to do so will cause damage. Some males can never fully retract their foreskin, therefore, force should never be used.

Hold the penis in the non-dominant hand, clean the prepuce in a circular motion.

If possible, retract the prepuce (some boys will have been circumcised, so this is not possible), and continue to clean the prepuce and glans in circular motions and using new gauze each time.

Rationale for catheterization

Urinary catheterization can be performed for a variety of reasons:
• Urinary retention
• Post-surgical procedures
• During acute illness to measure the urine output
• For diagnostic testing, such as urodynamics or micturating cystogram

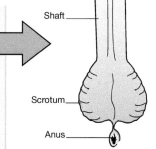

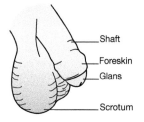

Children and Young People's Nursing Skills at a Glance, First Edition. Edited by Elizabeth Gormley-Fleming and Deborah Martin.
© 2018 John Wiley & Sons, Ltd. Published 2018 by John Wiley & Sons, Ltd.

Catheter insertion overview

Urinary catheterization is the insertion of a catheter into the bladder for the purpose of draining urine. It is an invasive procedure which should not be carried out without full consideration of all the presenting factors. Catheterization may be intermittent or continuous. As catheterization is associated with an increased risk of hospital-acquired infection, this is a sterile procedure.

Catheter selection

It is important that an appropriate catheter that is manufactured for the purpose of urinary catheterization is used. Catheters should conform to British Standards and the practice of using a polyvinyl chloride nasogastric tube as an alternative to a proper urinary catheter is discouraged. This non-recommended practice can cause harm to a patient.

Catheters come in a variety of lengths and diameter sizes, measured in Charriere (Ch) or French Gauge (Fg). Using an inappropriate size or length can cause trauma to the patient. Catheters of too large a diameter will cause irritation to the urethral mucosa and increase the possibility of a catheter-associated infection. The Foley indwelling catheter is the most commonly used and the table shows the recommended (Fg) sizes for the age of the child.

	Size of catheter (Fg)	
Age of child	Boys	Girls
0–5 months	6	6
6–12 months	6	6–8
1–3 years	8	8
4–7 years	10	10–12
8–12 years	12	12
Over 13 years	12–14	12–14

Consideration must also be given to the length of the catheter used and the size of the balloon to be inflated after insertion of the catheter.

Equipment

- Clean trolley
- Catheterization pack
- Catheter of appropriate size
- Catheter drainage system
- Disposable apron
- Sterile gloves
- Cleaning solution according to local policy, e.g. normal saline sachet, warmed in warm water
- Sterile gallipot and gauze swabs
- Sterile lubricant gel
- Lidocaine (local anaesthetic) gel
- Sterile water and syringe for filling balloon
- Adhesive strapping

Procedure

- Ask child to lie supine on the bed, maintain dignity by covering abdomen and lower legs.
- Place absorbent pad under the child's buttocks.
- To prevent cross-infection, put on apron and wash hands.
- Open catheter pack to provide sterile field.
- Apply hand gel, allow to hands to dry then put on sterile gloves.
- Open catheter, although leave in sterile inner sleeve, and put other equipment on to sterile field.
- Pour saline solution into gallipot.
- Put some lubricating gel onto a gauze swab and apply the nozzle to the lidocaine gel.
- Fill the syringe with sterile water ready to fill the catheter balloon.
- Tear the end of the plastic sleeve of the catheter to expose tip and apply lubricating lidocaine gel to the tip of the catheter, place in sterile bowl ready for use.
- Tear a hole in the sterile towel and place towel over child's groin area.
- Clean the child using gauze and normal saline.
- Apply the anaesthetic gel to the urethral meatus and wait 4 minutes for it to be effective.
- Change gloves, as the first pair are now contaminated.
- Insert the catheter into the urethra ensuring it does not touch any of the surrounding area.
- To prevent contamination, ensure the other end of the catheter remains in the plastic sleeve and in the sterile bowl.
- Once urine starts to flow, insert the catheter a further 2–4 cm. This will ensure that the balloon of the catheter is clear of the neck of the bladder, the balloon can be inflated without causing injury.
- Inflate the balloon with sterile water with the volume indicated on the catheter,
- Gently draw the catheter back until resistance is felt, the balloon is now sitting at the neck of the bladder.
- Attach urine drainage system to the end of the catheter, maintaining sterility to prevent contamination.
- Attach the catheter to the child's upper thigh to ensure there is no pull on the catheter which may cause trauma.
- Place the drainage bag on a hanger to keep the bag off the floor and below the level of the child's bladder.
- Reassure the child the procedure is over, clear away equipment in line with local policy.
- Consider if a urine sample needs to be sent.
- Wash and dry hands thoroughly.
- Document procedure in child's patient records.

Key points

- Read the label that is supplied with the catheter to identify the material, size, balloon capacity, and manufacturer's details prior to insertion.
- Preparation of the child is key to the successful insertion of a urinary catheter.
- Administer analgesia as required prior to the procedure.

43 Catheter care

Catheter care

A urinary catheter can be inserted into the bladder for the purpose of draining urine via the urethra or via the abdominal wall – suprapubic. Children's nurses have a responsibility to ensure they possess the required skills and keep themselves updated in line with evidenced-based practice to competently care for a child/young person with a urinary catheter.

The urinary system usually consists of two kidneys, two ureters, the bladder and the urethra. The kidneys filter waste products from the body and produces urine which is then drained via the ureters to the bladder where it is stored until voided via the urethra out of the body.

A child/young person may require a catheter if they have problems within the urinary system.

Reasons for catheterization may include:
• Retention of urine within the bladder.
• Urine drainage following surgery – this may be to promote healing after surgery of the renal system or for comfort following other major surgery.
• Accurate measurement of output in the very sick patient.
• For investigations such as a micturating cystogram.
• During end-of-life care.

A urethral catheter is passed via the urethra into the bladder; its position should be just inside the bladder but beyond the bladder neck to prevent injury. It is held in place with an inflatable balloon.

A suprapubic catheter is passed directly through the abdominal wall into the bladder. This procedure is generally carried out under general anaesthetic, although in life saving situations it may be inserted under local anaesthetic.

The catheter is attached to a urine drainage system to allow collection and measurement of the urine passed.

Anatomy of renal system

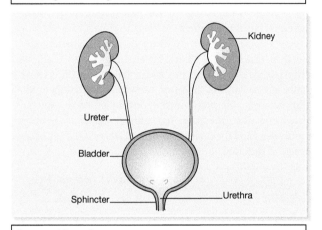

Suprapubic catheter

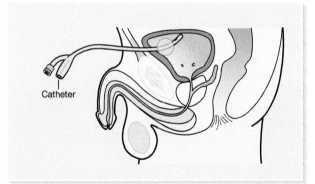

Urine bag drainage system

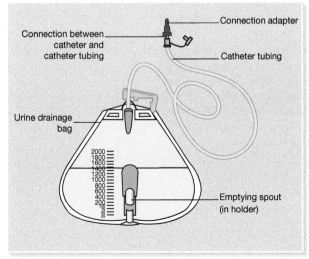

Urinary catheter in situ in bladder

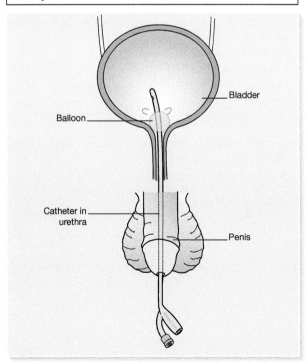

Children and Young People's Nursing Skills at a Glance, First Edition. Edited by Elizabeth Gormley-Fleming and Deborah Martin.
© 2018 John Wiley & Sons, Ltd. Published 2018 by John Wiley & Sons, Ltd.

Catheter care overview

Micro-organisms can enter the bladder during the insertion of the catheter or as a result of a catheter being in situ. The chance of infection increases each day that the catheter remains in situ. The two routes for micro-organisms to enter the bladder are:
• periurethral – between the outside of the catheter and the urethral wall;
• intraluminal – inside the catheter.

Once inside the bladder, micro-organisms may, in susceptible children, travel up the ureters to the kidney, causing kidney infection such as pyelonephritis.

Prevention of infection

• Good hygiene must be maintained and the urethral meatus (the entry to the urethra) should be washed daily with soap and water, strong perfumed soaps should be avoided. The use of antiseptic solutions to clean the meatus is not recommended. Washing should always occur from the front to the back in girls and in a circular motion for boys. A shallow bath is recommended for patients with suprapubic catheters.
• Cleaning of the catheter itself should be done from the urethral meatus down the catheter for a couple of centimetres.
• During daily washing the children's nurse should observe for signs of infection such as redness, swelling or any discharge.
• Urine drainage systems can also be a source of infection and they must always be suspended on a suitable stand, off the floor.
• Drainage bags should be emptied regularly (4-hourly) to allow urine to flow and prevent reflux of the urine back towards the child.
• When emptying the drainage bag, the tap should be cleaned inside and out with an alcohol swab and allowed to dry, to kill any micro-organisms that may be present and could then enter the drainage bag. Children's nurses must wear apron and gloves during this procedure.
• Ensuring an adequate or increased fluid intake and balanced diet will reduce the child's susceptibility to an infection.

General care principles

• Following insertion of a urethral catheter, the catheter should be securely held in place by taping the catheter to the abdomen or thigh. Regular checks should be made to ensure the catheter is not causing trauma to the urethral meatus.
• To ensure a good flow of urine, the drainage bag should be placed below the level of the child.
• The drainage system must remain kink-free at all times, do not allow the tube to get caught in the bed rails.

• The child's intake and output must be accurately recorded.
• When emptying the drainage bag, children's nurses should be aware of any signs of infection such as:
  • cloudy or foul-smelling urine;
  • the presence of protein/blood/leucocytes/nitrates on urinalysis.
• Regular observations of vital signs should be recorded. An increase in temperature may indicate an infection.
• Children and young people should also be regularly assessed for pain. Abdominal pain may indicate a urinary tract infection. Discomfort or pain at the urethral meatus may indicate trauma or infection. Children and young people may also experience bladder spasms as a result of the catheter irritating the bladder; these can be managed with the prescription of an anti-spasmodic medication.

Removal of a catheter

• Ensure the child or young person and family are suitably prepared for the removal of the catheter.
• Consider if analgesia is required prior to the procedure.
• Universal precautions must be adhered to.
• Remove the tape or strapping from the child's leg or abdomen using adhesive remover if necessary.
• Using an empty syringe, withdraw the water to deflate the balloon to the volume stated on the catheter. If the catheter has been in situ for a long time, some of the water may have leaked out.
• When the child is ready, hold the catheter near the entry site and gently using one steady motion, withdraw the catheter.
• Inspect the catheter to ensure it is intact and there are no signs of infection. Dispose of the catheter in line with Trust policy.
• Reassure the child or young person and advise that they may experience some discomfort in the next 24 hours. A warm bath can relieve this. Observe the child's urine output to ensure there is no retention or dysuria.
• Document the procedure and subsequent passing of urine in the patient's medical records.
• For suprapubic catheters, the retaining stitch is cut, the catheter withdrawn and pressure applied to the entry site for one minute to promote closure of the hole.

Key points

• Encourage an adequate fluid intake where permissible.
• Involve the child and family in caring for their catheter as much or as little as they wish.
• Normal personal hygiene habits can be maintained while the catheter is in situ.

44 Neurological assessment in children

Common causes of raised intracranial pressure

1. Cerebral oedema due to injury, infection, hypoxia

2. Cerebral haemorrhage

3. Meningitis/encephalitis

4. Space occupying lesion, i.e. tumour

5. Hydrocephalus

Required equipment

1. Neurological observation chart

2. Pen torch (not laser)

3. Blood pressure monitor

4. Oxygen saturation monitor

5. Thermometer

Glasgow Coma Scale (GCS) Teasdale and Jennett 1976

Glasgow Coma Scale		Score
Eye opening	Spontaneously	4
	To speech	3
	To pain	2
	None	1
Verbal response	Orientation	5
	Confusion	4
	Inappropriate	3
	Incomprehensible	2
	None	1
Motor response	Obeys commands	6
	Localizes to pain	5
	Withdraws from pain	4
	Flexion to pain	3
	Extension to pain	2
	None	1
Maximum score		15

Modified Glasgow Coma Scale for infants and children
Source: Reilly et al. (1988). Reproduced with permission of Springer

Glasgow Coma Scale	Child	Infant	Score
Eye opening	Spontaneous	Spontaneous	4
	To speech	To speech	3
	To pain	To pain	2
	No response	No response	1
Verbal response	Orientation, appropriate	Coos and babbles	5
	Confusion	Irritable cries	4
	Inappropriate words	Cries to pain	3
	Incomprehensible sounds	Moans to pain	2
	No response	No response	1
Motor response*	Obeys commands	Moves spontaneoeusly and purposefully	6
	Localizes painful stimulus	Withdraws to touch	5
	Withdraws in response to pain	Withdraws in response to pain	4
	Flexion in response to pain	Abnormal flexion posture to pain	3
	Extension in response to pain	Abnormal extension posture to pain	2
	No response	No response	1

*If patient is intubated, unconscious, or preverbal, the most important part of this scale is motor response. Motor response should be carefully evaluated.

Neurological assessment in children overview

Neurological assessment of children is a common nursing observation. It is primarily conducted for two reasons:
• to monitor a child with an altered level of consciousness after an event, e.g. after a convulsion;
• to monitor a child at risk of raised intracranial pressure following an event such as a head injury.
Neurological observations need to be performed when taking into account the child's developmental stage or any existing conditions that already impair a child's neurological function.

Family involvement

As with any observation in children, a full explanation should be given to both the child, in an age-appropriate manner, and the parents/carers. It is important to explain the reason for doing the observations and their frequency.

If English is not the child's first language, arrangements will need to be made to obtain a translator to help assess the child's neurological status.

Children and Young People's Nursing Skills at a Glance, First Edition. Edited by Elizabeth Gormley-Fleming and Deborah Martin.
© 2018 John Wiley & Sons, Ltd. Published 2018 by John Wiley & Sons, Ltd.

Equipment

Always collect all the required equipment prior to approaching the child and always observe the child from afar before coming close to him or her.

Primary assessment of neurological status

The quickest assessment of a child's level of consciousness is using the AVPU score:

A – **A**lert. Responsive, alert and orientated which means the child can identify people and is behaving normally.

V – Responds to **v**oice. This is often because a child is tired or in pain.

P – Responds only to **p**ain. Be careful when inflicting pain on children. Be sure to explain to the parents that this is necessary and use as little force as possible to obtain a response. Squeezing the trapezius or gently pulling a child's hair are among the kindest ways of inflicting pain.

U – Unresponsive. A child who is unresponsive or only responds to painful stimulus requires emergency treatment to protect his or her airway.

Secondary neurological assessment

It is recommended that the Glasgow Coma Scale (GCS) is used for the assessment of all children post head injury. GCS evaluates the child's ability to participate in three key activities: eye opening, verbal response and motor response.

Eye opening

Children post head injury will often refuse to open their eyes. Lights can be dimmed to reduce the glare distressing the child. Tempting a child to open their eyes to look at a TV screen or a toy is very effective.

Verbal response

Depending on the age of the child, obtaining a best verbal response is important. In a child who is talking, a verbal response should be appropriate and coherent. This can be done by asking three age-appropriate questions. Children can be talking but may be confused or disorientated and this is scored accordingly. In children who are not yet talking and babies, verbal sounds such as babbling can be reassuring. A high-pitched cry is a warning sign and can indicate raised intracranial pressure.

Motor response

Again, this assessment is age-specific. Ask the child to obey simple commands such as asking them stick out their tongue.

Pupil response

Pupil reaction is controlled by the third cranial nerve. The assessment looks at the following responses:

- brisk reaction: +
- no reaction: -
- sluggish reaction: S
- are the pupils equal and reacting to light (PEARL)?
- are the pupils dilated or pinpoint? This may indicate toxins.
- if one eye is closed, this is recorded as C.

Turn down the lights. Look into the eyes, are the pupils of equal size and shape? Shine a torch from the outer aspect of the eye towards the nose and observe the reaction of the pupil. Repeat on the other side.

Limb movement

It is important to look at all four limbs and to try to detect any weakness. See if the child can stand and walk, ask them to do this. If they cannot stand or they are too tired to stand, ask them to push your hands away with the soles of their feet. Squeezing your fingers and pushing your hands away can let you assess the strength of the upper limbs.

Posturing

Any abnormal posture can indicate severe neurological deficit

- opisthotonus – arching of the neck and back
- decorticate – arms are flexed/legs extended
- decerebrate – arms and legs are extended.

Physiological assessment

- Temperature, pulse, respirations, blood pressure and oxygen saturations are all recorded. Altered temperatures may indicate damage to the hypothalamus which regulates temperature. A slow bounding pulse, coupled with a rise in blood pressure, can indicate raised intracranial pressure.
- In children under 3, the unfused skull sutures can allow swelling to occur. In children under 18 months, always check for a bulging fontanelle.
- Always perform a blood glucose test on any unconscious child.
- Subtle changes in the assessment should be reported.
- Vomiting can be a sign of raised intracranial pressure and should be monitored and reported.

Who does the assessment and for how long?

There are advantages to having the same nurse carry out the observations over a period of time as then a rapport can be built up with both the child and carer.

The frequency of observation will depend on the situation of the child. Any abnormal observation should increase the frequency to every 15 minutes. In a well child, this can range from 30 minutes to hourly.

Carrying out neurological observations at night can be very challenging with both child and parent/carer becoming irritable but it is necessary. It is important to explain this to the family before they go to sleep.

Documentation

All neurological observations should be recorded on a neurological observation chart. Any changes should be discussed with the nurse in charge and a doctor.

Key points

- Neurological observations in children can be challenging to perform and upsetting for the child and family.
- Identifying abnormalities during the assessment can prevent catastrophic damage to a child.
- The normal behaviour for the child must be known in order to make a holistic and accurate assessment of their neurological status.
- At handover, it is best practice if the nurse taking over the care of the child and the nurse who has been caring for the child complete a set of neurological observations together.

References

British Paediatric Neurology Association (2004) Available at: https://www.bpna.org.uk/

Reilly, P.L. et al. (1988) Assessing the conscious level in infants and young children: a paediatric version of the Glasgow Coma Scale. *Child's Nervous System*, 4(1), 30–33.

Teasdale, G. and Jennett, B. (1976) Assessment and prognosis of coma after head injury. *Acta Neurology Supplement*. 34, 45–55.

45 Preparation for a lumbar puncture

Position of child for lumbar puncture

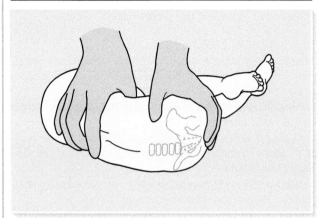

Collection of CSF and position of spinal needle

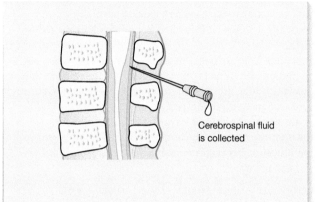

Cerebrospinal fluid
is collected

Subarachnoid space

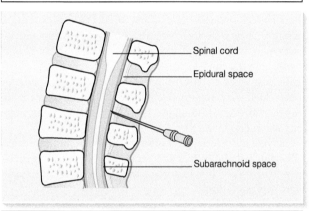

Spinal cord

Epidural space

Subarachnoid space

Collecting CSF

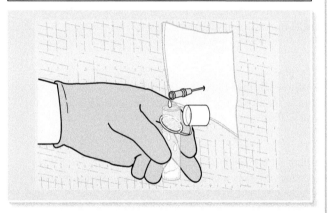

Lumbar puncture needle size

Age of child	Height of child (cm)	Size of needle (length) (cm)
Preterm neonate	< 50	2
< 2 years	50–80	3
2–5 years	80–120	4
5–12 years	120–150	5
> 12 years	150–180	6

Preparation for a lumbar puncture overview

A lumbar puncture is an invasive procedure that involves the insertion of a needle into the subarachnoid space. This will be performed to assist with diagnosis or to permit treatment. For diagnostic purposes, a sample of the cerebrospinal fluid (CSF) is taken if meningitis, encephalitis or other neurological conditions are suspected. It may also be used to remove excess CSF and measure the pressure of the CSF. Contrast media may also be inserted into the subarachnoid space during radiological investigation. Medication may be instilled when a lumbar puncture is required for therapeutic purposes.

An invasive and high-risk procedure, this must be performed aseptically and by an experienced doctor. Two nurses are required to assist with this procedure.

Written consent should be obtained.

Role of the nurse

The role of the nurse in a lumbar puncture is to provide a safe environment in which the procedure may be performed. Supporting the child and family is essential at all stages. The nurse who assumes the responsibility of positioning the child during the lumbar puncture must understand the safe holding technique and be fully conversant with the potential contraindications and complications of this procedure. The nurse who is assisting the doctor needs to understand the principles of aseptic technique and adhere to this when assisting with a lumbar puncture.

Equipment

Lumbar puncture pack
Lumbar puncture needles correct size
Sterile cleaning agent
Sterile containers × 3
Glucose sample container
Specimen request form
Sterile towels
Sterile gloves
Local anaesthetic
Sterile adhesive dressing
Local policy must be adhered to in regard to skin cleansing agent and collection containers used.

If the child is sedated or seriously ill, then monitoring equipment must be in situ.

Procedure

• Prepare the equipment
• Nurse 1: Position the child, right or left side on the edge of the examination bed. Knees are drawn up towards chest and neck is flexed. Craniospinalaxis is parallel to the bed. This position will need to be maintained for the duration of the procedure.
• It is useful to have play specialist available to talk to child and provide distraction during procedure.
• Nurse 2: Remove the local anaesthetic cream and assist the doctor in cleaning the skin and administering the local anaesthetic.
• Doctor will insert the needle between L3 and L4 or L4 and L5.
• Discard the first few drops of CSF.
• Collect 1–2 ml (10 drops maximum) in each sterile container. Label 1, 2, 3 in order of collection.
• Apply sterile dressing to puncture site once needle has been removed.
• Safely dispose of all equipment.
• Observe puncture site for CSF leakage and ask the child if they have any headache.
• Encourage the child to lie flat if possible, adhere to local guidelines.
• Record vital signs and neurological observations if indicated.
• Report all abnormalities in vital signs, behaviour or CSF leakage immediately.
• Administer analgesia as prescribed post procedure.
• Maintain nursing records as required.
• Keep family and child informed of results and implications of these.

Side-effects of a lumbar puncture

• Headache
• CSF leak from puncture site
• Back pain at site
• Bleeding from puncture site
• Herniation of cerebrum
• Infection.

Key points
• A lumbar puncture is contraindicated in the presence of raised intracranial pressure.
• Correct positioning of the child is essential.
• Avoid over-flexing the neck as it may lead to respiratory compromise.
• Strict asepsis is required at every stage of the procedure.

46 Neurovascular assessment

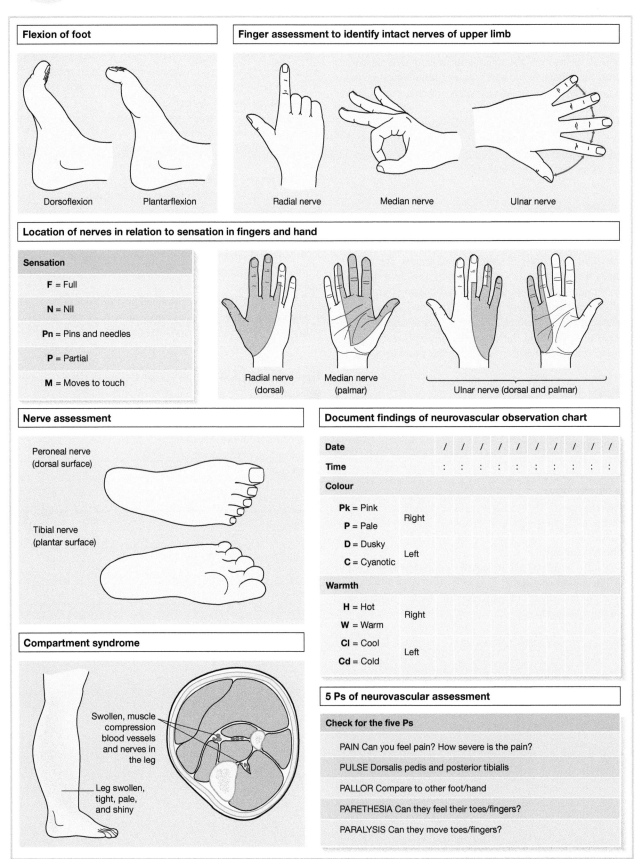

Flexion of foot

Dorsoflexion   Plantarflexion

Finger assessment to identify intact nerves of upper limb

Radial nerve   Median nerve   Ulnar nerve

Location of nerves in relation to sensation in fingers and hand

Sensation

F = Full

N = Nil

Pn = Pins and needles

P = Partial

M = Moves to touch

Radial nerve (dorsal)   Median nerve (palmar)   Ulnar nerve (dorsal and palmar)

Nerve assessment

Peroneal nerve (dorsal surface)

Tibial nerve (plantar surface)

Compartment syndrome

Swollen, muscle compression blood vessels and nerves in the leg

Leg swollen, tight, pale, and shiny

Document findings of neurovascular observation chart

Date	/	/	/	/	/	/	/	/	/	/
Time	:	:	:	:	:	:	:	:	:	:
Colour										

Pk = Pink
P = Pale — Right
D = Dusky
C = Cyanotic — Left

Warmth

H = Hot
W = Warm — Right
Cl = Cool
Cd = Cold — Left

5 Ps of neurovascular assessment

Check for the five Ps

PAIN Can you feel pain? How severe is the pain?

PULSE Dorsalis pedis and posterior tibialis

PALLOR Compare to other foot/hand

PARETHESIA Can they feel their toes/fingers?

PARALYSIS Can they move toes/fingers?

Children and Young People's Nursing Skills at a Glance, First Edition. Edited by Elizabeth Gormley-Fleming and Deborah Martin.
© 2018 John Wiley & Sons, Ltd. Published 2018 by John Wiley & Sons, Ltd.

Neurovascular assessment overview

Neurovascular observations are an essential part of the infant's or child's care if they present with an orthopaedic condition in order to avoid the development of Compartment syndrome, which can lead to devastating consequences. If any neurovascular compromise is detected, then prompt treatment is required.

Neurovascular assessment requires a thorough assessment of the fingers or toes on the affected limb. This assessment involves checking the 5 Ps.

- **Pain**
- **Pulse**
- **Pallor**
- **Paresthesia**
- **Paralysis**

Pain

Using an appropriate pain assessment tool, pain should be at the fracture site and not elsewhere. Analgesia should be given as prescribed and monitored for effectiveness.

Pulses

Radial, dorsalis pads and posterior tibialis should be assessed and grade noted. Again comparison should be made with the unaffected limb. A Doppler may be used.

Colour

The fingers or toes should be normal skin tone. Any deviation from this is suggestive of an inadequate blood flow. Comparison should be made with the unaffected limb. White, purple or blue colour is indicative of compromised blood flow.

Sensation

There should be normal sensation. Numbness and tingling (paresthesia) are not normal and may be present initially post injury or surgery due to nerve trauma. The nerve affected will be identified by the altered sensation in the relevant finger or toe. Sensation should be recorded as normal, reduced, pins and needles, partial, or moves to touch.

Movement

The child should be able to flex, extend and abduct their foot, hand, fingers and toes. This may be restricted by the plaster of Paris or the cast. Thumb-finger opposition should be present. The infant is not going to co-operate so passive assessment should be carried out.

Other indicators to be checked are:

Warmth

Compare with the unaffected digits, they should both be the same temperature when touched. If the digits are cool, then identify possible reason. How long since surgery? Is plaster of Paris still wet? Is limb exposed to the cool room temperature?

Capillary refill time

This should be <2 seconds in the digits of the affected limb. Ambient room temperature should be considered. The nail bed should be compressed for the count of 5. Normal colour should return within 2 seconds. Any time longer than this is suggestive of circulatory compromise.

Swelling

Some swelling is likely post trauma and surgery but the skin should not be shiny or taut. The limb should be elevated either by tilting the bed/cot for a lower limb or using a Bradford Sling or pillows for an upper limb injury.

Plaster/cast

Check around both top and bottom to ensure they are not too tight.

All findings should be clearly documented on the neurovascular assessment chart. The severity of the injury and type of surgery will dictate the frequency of the neurovascular assessment.

Key points
- Very young children and pre-verbal children will not be able to answer questions or obey commands, so this makes neurovascular assessment more difficult.
- Pain and fear may prevent the child from co-operating, particularly when asked to move or wriggle their fingers/toes.
- If any concerns are identified during neurovascular assessment, then the orthopaedic team or relevant team should be contacted in case Compartment syndrome is developing.

47 Care of a cast

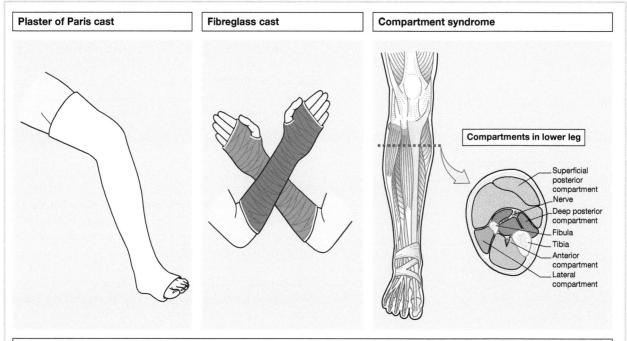

| Plaster of Paris cast | Fibreglass cast | Compartment syndrome |

Compartments in lower leg

- Superficial posterior compartment
- Nerve
- Deep posterior compartment
- Fibula
- Tibia
- Anterior compartment
- Lateral compartment

Plaster of Paris vs fibreglass

Plaster of Paris	Advantages
Used mainly for new fractures	Stronger, pliable
Following surgery when bleeding is likely	Easy to mould, ensuring smoothing to conform to the bone
	May be split easily, to enable room for swelling
	More malleable
	Cheaper financially
	Worldwide usage
Fibreglass/polyurethane	Advantages
Fibreglass	Light but sturdy
Used for stabilization following initial injury	Coloured bandages giving the child a choice, thereby engaging the child in their cast
As an add-on extra top layer of colour	Dries within 30 minutes

Advice on discharge: 'do's for child and parents

Keep plaster dry. If it does start to crumble, attend plaster department or A/E for reinforcement of the cast

Keep the limb elevated, using a sling or cushions

Keep moving limb or toes/fingers hourly

Take simple analgesia

Observe the limb for swelling/discoloration/altered sensation/excess pain especially on stretching the digits/tightness of the plaster

Attend plaster department or A/E if worried

Advice on discharge: 'don't's for child and parents

DO NOT get the plaster wet or moist

DO NOT keep the limb hanging down

DO NOT put anything down inside the plaster

DO NOT cut/damage the plaster

DO NOT weight bear unless told to do so

DO NOT lean the limb against anything

DO NOT dry the plaster with a hairdryer or heater

Children and Young People's Nursing Skills at a Glance, First Edition. Edited by Elizabeth Gormley-Fleming and Deborah Martin.
© 2018 John Wiley & Sons, Ltd. Published 2018 by John Wiley & Sons, Ltd.

Care of a cast overview
Types of cast

A plaster cast is an open weave bandage which is impregnated with gypsum and when wet and applied to a limb, sets hard. It is commonly called a plaster of Paris. It is soaked in warm water before application and starts to set in 5 minutes. It takes up to 48 hours to dry, hence it can be damaged if it is not moulded and applied with the palms of the hand. Before it dries completely, it should not rest against a hard or sharp surface as it will cause damage.

A fibreglass plaster is a knitted bandage which is impregnated with a resin structure. It sets within minutes of being wet, and dries within 30 minutes, which allows light weight-bearing quickly. It does, however, need up to 8 layers for sturdiness. Once applied, the fibreglass plaster will have sharp edges which needs to be covered by elastoplast or sleek to prevent skin damage. The limb must be in the correct position before application, as due to its rapid setting time it is not as easily moulded. The plasters are popular with the child/parents as they are lighter, and can be made into a coloured form, which the child can choose, thereby giving them some input into their care.

Structure of a cast

There are times when a combination of plasters are used, with the outer layer being the coloured one. Each plaster has a stockinette and wool bandage applied prior to application. The wool bandage protects the fracture and has extra layers over bony prominences.

Newly applied casts of whichever material must be left to dry naturally. Using drying aids, such as a heater or a hair dryer, will cause damage to the plaster, but more importantly the plaster conducts heat which may cause the skin to burn. However, both plasters will feel warm after application, due to the chemical reaction. This may be a comfort to the child, but it is essential to inform the child and family of this phenomenon.

It is important to elevate the limb after application for 48 hours to prevent swelling. If pillows are used to elevate, a towel under the plaster will absorb any moisture.

'Do's and 'don't's with a plaster cast

- Elevate the limb for at least 48+ hours on pillows/cushions, or use a sling.
- Do not weight bear unless instructed to do so.
- Do not lean or rest on a sharp edge.
- Keep the plaster cast dry at all times. If it becomes wet/moist, it will crumble or crack, which will not allow it to provide the support needed.
- Do not poke anything down the cast, or put any object down the cast.
- If it itches, massage the outside of the plaster, which will help.

A simple advice card with essential advice is given to the parents and carers and will allow them to care with confidence while at home, and know when to seek medical help.

Compartment syndrome

Compartment syndrome can occur when the neurovascular system becomes compromised by pressure on the nerves or blood vessels, which can damage the circulation, and compress the nerves. If it is not dealt with immediately, there will be damage to these structures, causing loss of tissue, loss of movement and feeling, and, in the worst case scenario, loss of the limb.

While the child is hospitalized, the staff must perform circulation observations hourly to recognize and prevent compartment syndrome. Explain to the parents why the limb is being assessed, and teach them to observe it at home. If there is any doubt about the integrity of the limb, the doctor must be informed immediately. Documentation of these observations is essential.

Key points
- The neurovascular status of the toes or fingers must be checked regularly and findings documented.
- Any alteration to circulation distal to the cast must be reported to the medical staff at once.
- Encourage the child to wriggle their toes and fingers as much as possible while in the cast.

48 Skin traction

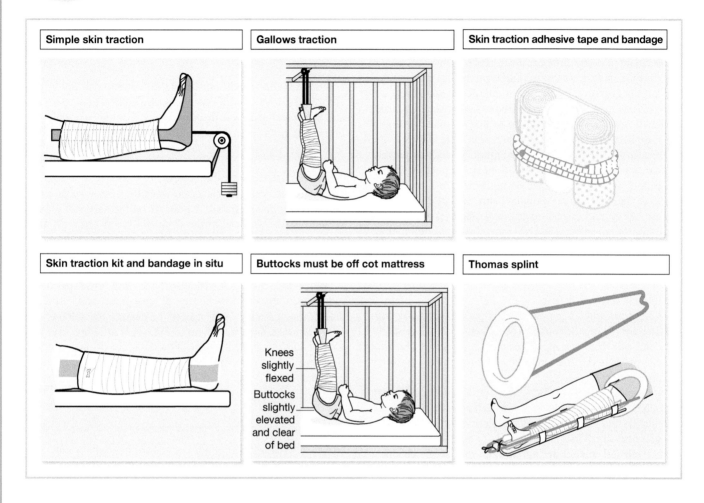

| Simple skin traction | Gallows traction | Skin traction adhesive tape and bandage |

| Skin traction kit and bandage in situ | Buttocks must be off cot mattress | Thomas splint |

Knees slightly flexed

Buttocks slightly elevated and clear of bed

Skin traction overview

Traction is used for various conditions which affect children. It is a pulling force through power; the application of a sustained pull on a limb/muscle maintains the position of a fractured bone, or corrects a deformity.

Reasons for traction

• Stabilization and maintenance of position of a limb.
• Rest and immobilization of a limb which is affected by trauma or infection such as septic arthritis.
• Pain relief from irritable hip/slipped upper femoral epiphyses.
• Correction of orthopaedic conditions which may be congenital, e.g. hip dysplasia, or acquired, e.g. Perthes disease, which is a hip disorder.
• Alleviation of muscle spasm, e.g. locked knee.
• Prior to surgery, to allow a joint to be relieved of its pressure, e.g. the ball and socket joint where the head of the bone is pulled away from its socket as in the hip/shoulder joint.
Children of all ages may at some time in their lives require a period of bed rest for the application of traction to assist in alleviating their condition.

Types of traction

• *Fixed*: The pull is applied between two fixed points, e.g. a fractured femur where the skin extension tape cords are tied to the end of the splint or the bed. The counter-pressure is exerted by the ring of a Thomas splint against the ischial tuberosity of the pelvis.
• *Balanced traction*: This is the pull between weights attached to the end of the skin extension tapes, with the counter-traction applied by the child's weight, such as in Pugh's traction.

Application types

• *Gallows*: Modified gallows/hoop traction is used in the treatment of hip dysplasia for babies, or to treat babies/toddlers with a fractured shaft femur (for a child below 2–14 kg approximately). This traction allows the hips to be abducted to a maximum 60 degrees, post 24 hours application. It should not be used for longer than 3–4 weeks. Gallows traction is advantageous for a child who may be nursed at home, if there is a children's community team specialized in orthopaedic conditions available and can visit daily.
• *Pugh's traction*: This is a kind of straight leg traction and is used in the following situations: in pre-operative conditions,

Children and Young People's Nursing Skills at a Glance, First Edition. Edited by Elizabeth Gormley-Fleming and Deborah Martin.
© 2018 John Wiley & Sons, Ltd. Published 2018 by John Wiley & Sons, Ltd.

e.g. in slipped upper femoral epiphyses (SUFE); post-operatively to allow the joint to heal following hip/knee surgery; if there is infection in a joint; in Perthes disease and to rest/immobilize the joint.

Applying balanced traction

Balanced traction is generally applied following trauma when the child is very agitated with pain and fear. Prior to application, it is essential to consider the expertise of the staff, the child's needs at the time, the choice of equipment, and the pre- and post-application needs. An assessment must be carried out before the application as to whether the child will need analgesia/sedation, or Entonox for the procedure.

Whenever traction is applied, it is essential that staff have the expertise to apply the traction safely, and this would include a play therapist to aid distraction; Equipment must be prepared including attachment of a balkan beam frame, if necessary. An important part of the application is a thorough explanation of the procedure, including the reasons for it and the approximate time it will be necessary to leave the child in traction, bearing in mind the child's cognition, and consent for the procedure from both child and parents/carer.

Types of extension tapes

There are two types of extension tapes:
- *adhesive*: used in gallows/hoop/balanced traction
- *non-adhesive*: used in Pugh's/simple straight leg traction

If the tapes are to stay attached for more than one week, then adhesive tape is preferable. If the tapes are to be removed more than once a day, consider using non-adhesive tape. However, if the child is restless and cannot tolerate the frequent application and removal, consider using adhesive tape. Whichever is used, it must be appropriate for the treatment.

Equipment

- Skin adhesive spray: to enhance adherence when using adhesive tapes
- Tapes
- Bandages
- Weights held in a cradle for safety
- Splints
- Extra cord
- Bed that can be elevated at the foot end, and any other equipment that the bed may need, such as balkan beams
- Hoops.

If a Thomas splint is to be used, measuring the upper thigh will help to determine the size of the ring. Measuring the circumference of the good thigh at its widest part and adding extra centimetres to allow for swelling, which can be caused by internal bleeding, bruising, and the irregularity of the bones, will be necessary to achieve the correct size. This is also the correct time to examine the skin for any integrity such as wounds. Ensure the documentation includes the size of splint, the type of extension tapes, the skin integrity and the sedation or analgesia given.

Procedure

- Measure from the maleoli to the upper thigh or tibial tuberosity on both sides. Ensure that all bony prominences have padding to cover them.
- When using adhesive tapes, peel the plaster back as you are applying it, to prevent wrinkles which may cause skin damage.
- When applying the outer bandage, keep the knee free, begin at the maleoli, leaving the foot free and do not apply too tightly.
- Weights: ensure the correct sizes are put in a safety cradle, and are not too heavy, which would cause the counter-production of balanced traction. Ensure the child is lying flat, so that the weights will not rest on the floor when the child is sleeping.
- Attach the cord to the weights, ensuring they are taped safely to their harness, to prevent them falling off and causing injury.
- Elevate the foot of the bed to ensure counter-balance.
- If the tapes are attached to a hoop or gallows frame, ensure there is a hand-free area under the child's bottom to provide the traction.

Post-application care

- Neurovascular observations: 1–4 hourly to prevent risk of compartment syndrome.
- Ensure the adherence of the tapes twice daily, and observe the tissue integrity.
- Analgesia: an anti-spasmodic may be considered by the medical team.
- Physiotherapist input for prevention of muscle wastage, foot drop and to provide muscle exercises.
- Distraction and play involvement.
- Holistic care.
- Dietician involvement.
- Bowels/urine recording.

Key points

- Pressure area care is essential as skin integrity may be interrupted particularly under the adhesive skin extensions.
- Infants and toddlers nursed on gallows traction may be prone to choking, so extreme care must be taken with feeding.

49 SteriStrip™ application

Clean wound using aseptic technique

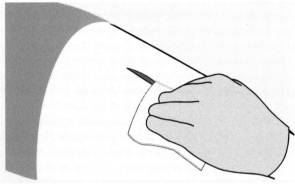

Remove card and maintain sterile field, bend card at end perforation and gently remove tab

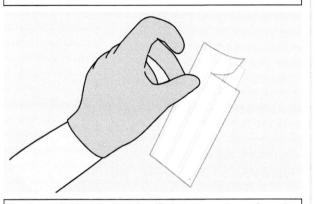

Grasp end of skin closure strip with a gloved hand or foreceps and peel off card

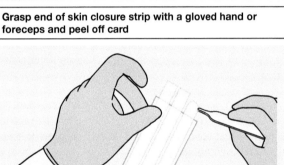

Apply one half of the first SteriStrip to wound margin and press firmly in place

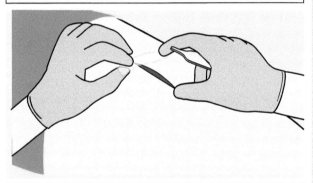

Press free half of SteriStrip firmly on other side of the wound

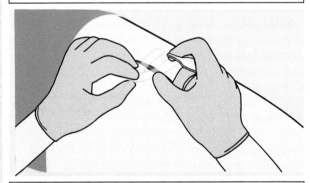

The rest of the wound should be closed with additional SteriStrip

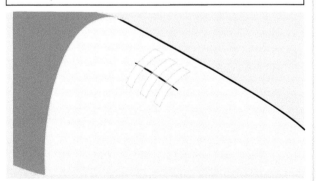

Additional SteriStrips can be placed vertically over all edges of the applied SteriStrip to reinforce the closure

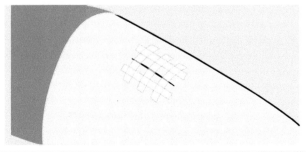

Children and Young People's Nursing Skills at a Glance, First Edition. Edited by elizabeth Gormley-Fleming and Deborah Martin.
© 2018 John Wiley & Sons, Ltd. Published 2018 by John Wiley & Sons, Ltd.

SteriStrip application overview

SteriStrips are small sticky strips used for wound closure. They come in a variety of lengths and widths to suit different wounds. There are different types of wound closure strips available such as SteriStrips or Leukostrips™, both of these are trade names. These are very similar in nature except SteriStrips are made out of paper and Leukostrips are made of material. Leukostrips are preferred in practice as they adhere to the skin better and allow a small amount of stretch in the strip, thus making them more flexible. Wound closure strips are preferable to using sutures, as this is a quick, relatively painless procedure and much less distressing for children.

When to use SteriStrips

SteriStrips can be used on most wounds all over the body, providing the underlying structures are intact. Areas that should be avoided are the lips, in the scalp and in the hair and the eyebrows. SteriStrips should not be applied to the lips as this is an area that easily becomes moist and wet. Large lip wounds and wounds that pass through the vermilion border should be assessed by the plastics team. SteriStrips should not be applied in the hair or eyebrows as they will not be able to stick effectively.

Due to the large numbers of movements that joints perform, SteriStrips are not always able to hold large wounds closed over a big joint such as knees or elbows. Depending on the size of the wound, you may be able to SteriStrip the wound with the joint in a flexed position. This allows the SteriStrips to be applied when the skin is stretched so when the joint is flexed, the SteriStrips are maintained in position.

How to select the right size of SteriStrips

The larger the wound, the larger the SteriStrip required. Longer SteriStrips allow for more tension to be applied to the wound, so when closing a very large or open wound, these will help to hold the wound closed. SteriStrips may have to be cut to suit small wounds or small areas of skin.

How to apply SteriStrips

Young children may need to be held still by a parent so that the wound can be closed quickly and effectively. The use of distraction can help make the procedure easier and less distressing for the child. Always ensure the child has had adequate pain relief before the procedure takes place as cleaning the wound may be uncomfortable.

Once the wound has been assessed and cleaned, using a non-touch aseptic technique, the SteriStrips are safe to be applied. While cleaning, assess the wound to make sure the edges of the wound come together nicely. Sterile scissors must be used to trim any adipose tissue that cannot be reinserted back into the wound. Any trimming should be minimal as further bleeding should be avoided.

Procedure

- Remove the card using sterile precautions as necessary.
- Bend card at the end perforation and gently remove tab.
- Grasp end of skin closure strip with a gloved hand or forceps and peel off the card.
- Apply one half of the first SteriStrip to the wound margin and press it firmly in place.
- Using fingers or forceps, appose skin edges as closely as possible.
- Press free half of SteriStrip firmly on other side of the wound.
- The rest of the wound should be closed with additional SteriStrips until all the wound edges are closed. Additional SteriStrips can be placed vertically over all edges of the applied SteriStrips to reinforce the closure.
- If you are not happy with the closure, SteriStrips can be peeled back and replaced.

Care of SteriStrips

SteriStrips need to be kept clean and dry to ensure they stay intact. They should be left open to the air with no extra dressing if possible to prevent further infection. Small children may require extra dressings to ensure the SteriStrips stay in place.

SteriStrips should be left on for 5–7 days, depending on the depth and severity of the wound. After this time, they can be soaked off in the bath.

The wound should be observed regularly for any signs of infection. If the wound becomes red, hot to touch, or develops any odour, medical attention should be sought and antibiotics considered.

Key points
- The wound must be cleaned prior to applying SteriStrips
- Areas that are likely to get wet, e.g. chin and areas with sweat, should be avoided and another method for wound closure identified.

50 Wet wrapping in atopic eczema

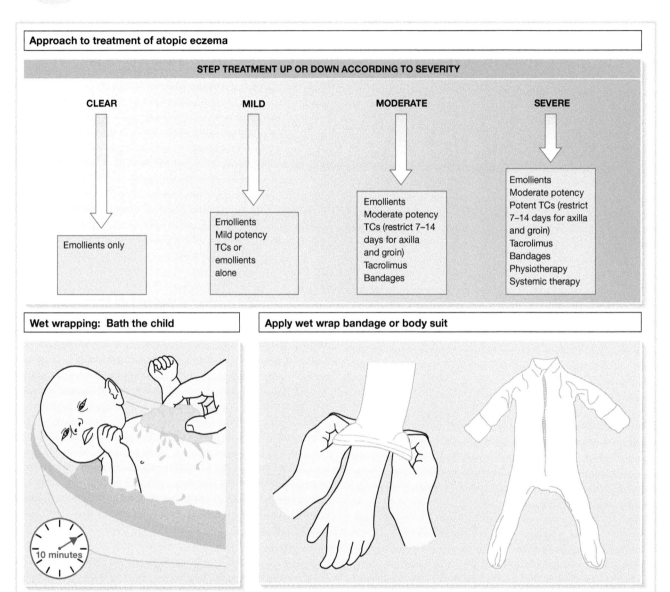

Approach to treatment of atopic eczema

STEP TREATMENT UP OR DOWN ACCORDING TO SEVERITY

CLEAR

Emollients only

MILD

Emollients
Mild potency
TCs or
emollients
alone

MODERATE

Emollients
Moderate potency
TCs (restrict 7–14
days for axilla
and groin)
Tacrolimus
Bandages

SEVERE

Emollients
Moderate potency
Potent TCs (restrict
7–14 days for axilla
and groin)
Tacrolimus
Bandages
Physiotherapy
Systemic therapy

Wet wrapping: Bath the child

10 minutes

Apply wet wrap bandage or body suit

Wet wrapping overview

Wet wraps are a bandaging technique that may be used as part of treatment for moderate to severe atopic eczema. Wet wrapping is believed to work by evaporation, rehydration and protection.

Atopic eczema management

Healthcare professionals should use a stepped approach to manage atopic eczema in children. This means tailoring the treatment step to the severity of the atopic eczema. Emollients should form the basis of atopic eczema management and should always be used, even when the atopic eczema is clear. Management can then be stepped up or down, according to the severity of symptoms, with the addition of the other treatments.

Healthcare professionals should offer children with atopic eczema and their parents/carers information on how to recognize flares of atopic eczema (increased dryness, itching, and redness, swelling and general irritability). They should give clear instructions on how to manage flares according to the stepped-care plan, and prescribe treatments that allow children and their parents or carers to follow this plan.

Frequent and generous use of emollients helps the skin to feel more comfortable and less itchy. They keep the skin moist and flexible, helping to prevent cracks. Emollients are available as creams, ointments and lotions, any or all of which might be suitable to use at different times, depending on whether a person's eczema reacts to a specific ingredient in an emollient. When applying emollients, in order to prevent contamination of bacteria from the skin to the cream, it is vital that you do not use your hands to apply the emollient. The cream should be removed from the tub with a clean spatula/spoon.

Topical corticosteroids in atopic eczema

Topical corticosteroids (TCs) block some of the effects of the chemicals used by the immune system to trigger the process of inflammation, and make the immune system less sensitive, meaning it is less likely to cause symptoms that affect the skin. They help to regulate the production of new skin cells and narrow the blood vessels in the affected areas of skin, thus reducing the amount of inflammatory chemicals sent to the skin. Topical steroid preparations are divided into four categories according to how strong or potent they are: mild, moderately potent, potent and very potent. The potency of topical corticosteroids should be tailored to the severity of the child's atopic eczema, which may vary according to body site.

Potency of topical corticosteroids
- Use mild potency for mild atopic eczema.
- Use moderate potency for moderate atopic eczema.
- Use potent TCs for severe atopic eczema
- Use mild potency for the face and neck, except for short-term (3–5 days) use of moderate potency for severe flares.

Fear of side effects can make people under-treat their eczema by stopping treatment too soon or not using the steroid they have been given. This can affect the overall management of the condition and may mean that a stronger preparation has to be used to bring the eczema under control again. If potent topical steroids are used for a long period of time, particularly to the face and flexures, without adequate supervision, skin thinning can occur. If atopic eczema is not controlled by topical corticosteroids and if there is risk of important adverse effects from topical corticosteroid treatment, then treatment with topical calcineurin inhibitors should be considered. These are immune-modulatory drugs, which means it modulates or changes the immune system to reduce skin inflammation.

Treatment using wet wrapping

Wet wraps are particularly useful for children with moderate to severe eczema whose skin is not made comfortable with the sole application of moisturizers and appropriate topical steroids. A particular indication for wet wrapping is severe night-time itching where the family is kept awake by the child's inability to sleep due to the cycle of itching and scratching.

An emollient or topical steroid should be applied to the skin after the bath and before the inner layer of the wet wrap is applied to the skin. The inner layer is soaked in warm tap water and gently squeezed out before being applied to the trunk and limbs. The wet layer is applied first and the dry layer is folded back on itself to cover the hands and feet. The wraps create a warm humid environment, which encourages bacterial growth, and this can spread the infection. They should therefore not be used in the visible presence of any bacterial, fungal or viral infection.

The advantages of wet wrapping are:
- *Evaporation*: The gradual drying out of the wet layer has a cooling effect on the skin, therefore reducing itching and discomfort. It is therefore essential that the bandages are remoistened and not allowed to completely dry out.
- *Rehydration*: This is putting moisture back into the skin. The skin absorbs the large amount of emollient used and so in general will soften the skin, when a wet wrap is used.
- *Protection*: The body suit puts a barrier between the child's fingers and the skin, thus reducing any damage to the skin caused by scratching and so encourages the damaged skin to heal.

Key points
- The wet wrapping should be used for short-term treatment only.
- Bandages must be secured correctly to prevent the child from unwrapping them.

51 12-lead electrocardiography

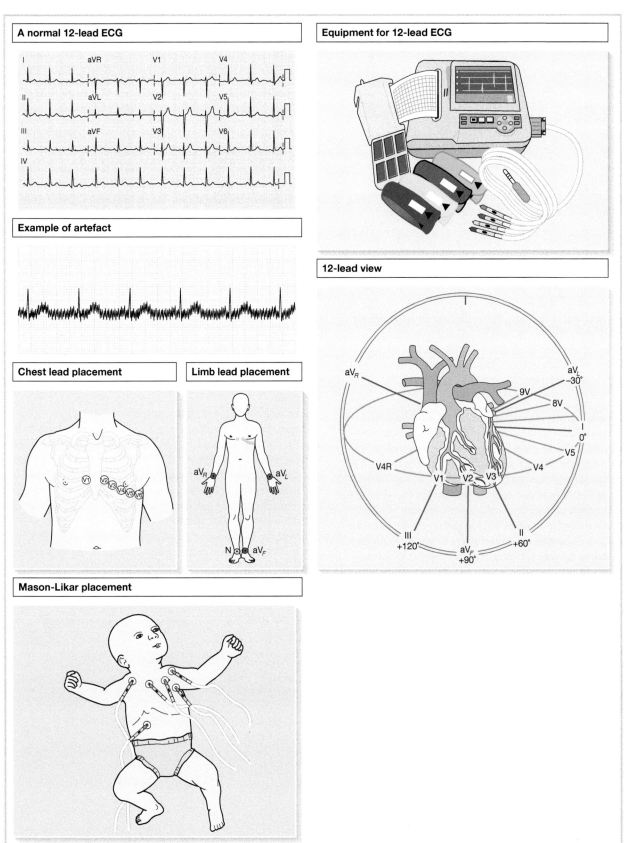

A normal 12-lead ECG

Example of artefact

Chest lead placement

Limb lead placement

Mason-Likar placement

Equipment for 12-lead ECG

12-lead view

Children and Young People's Nursing Skills at a Glance, First Edition. Edited by Elizabeth Gormley-Fleming and Deborah Martin.
© 2018 John Wiley & Sons, Ltd. Published 2018 by John Wiley & Sons, Ltd.

12-lead electrocardiography overview

Taking a 12-lead ECG reading from a child or infant can be either a quick process with minimal fuss, or equally, it can be very stressful for the patient, their family or carer and the person performing the procedure. It is common for infants in particular to cry when they are undressed and cold, this can be problematic as this can cause an 'artefact' reading in the recording and reduce its value. By being as prepared and swift as possible, the outcome is likely to be better. It can be the case that a recording is simply too difficult due to an infant or child becoming too distressed. In the situation where distress could precipitate a crisis or collapse, it is best to stop and try later, relying on other clinical signs for information in the meantime. As the patient's advocate, it is important to remain mindful of the whole child and if distress is likely to compromise the child, then stop the procedure.

Preparation

As younger children and infants often find it scary being cold and having to lie still and become upset as a consequence, ensure all equipment is checked (plugged in or has sufficient charge) before commencing. Check the date and time are correct on the machine and that there is sufficient ECG paper and electrodes (at least 20). Ensure the electrodes are in date and appear sticky – they become less conductive with less adhesion. When this is all correct, then confirm the patient's identity – request the patient's full name and date of birth and check the procedure to be performed and obtain consent from the child, young person or their parent/carer. Ensure the patient is in the supine position if possible. If the patient is restless and distressed, the procedure may be performed with the patient in a sitting position, although this may give a poorer quality reading. Skin is a poor conductor of electricity, therefore good skin preparation is important; clean the skin, exfoliate if necessary with light abrasion using abrasive tape if adhesion is difficult or the skin has recently been moisturized – care should be taken in patients with sensitive or broken skin as this may aggravate their skin. Ensure the patient is relaxed and comfortable in order to reduce artefact, ensure visual confirmation of an artefact-free ECG trace on the display before pressing the appropriate record or print button on the ECG machine to obtain a resting 12-lead ECG reading.

Settings and artefact

Record a 12-lead ECG at 25 mm/sec with a gain setting of 10 mm/m unless instructed otherwise, for example, increasing the gain if the complexes are of a low voltage. This may be the case due to a number of clinical issues – if the recording appears low in voltage, take note of this and inform the person reading the ECG, this information could be critical. Ensure any change in gain is clearly marked on the printed ECG recording. If artefact remains, consider sources other than muscle tremor, for example, medical equipment or mobile phones. If it is safe to do so, turn off any equipment that may be causing the artefact. If you are unsure about the safety, check!

Application of the leads

Despite being called a 12-lead ECG trace, it only involves 10 leads (but gives a view 12 ways). Positioning and accuracy are important as information is derived on the presumption that the leads are correctly placed. Regarding infants and younger children, standard chest and limb lead placements apply. However, if they are particularly distressed, the Mason-Likar lead placement can be used. Limb electrodes are placed anteriorly on the left and right shoulder and left and right side of the lower torso to reduce artefact caused by the movement of the limbs.

Electrode position: limb leads

The position of the electrodes for the limb leads is shown in the Figure:
RA (Right arm): Right forearm, proximal to the wrist.
LA (Left arm): Left forearm, proximal to the wrist.
LL (Left leg): Left lower leg, proximal to the ankle.
RL (Right leg): Right lower leg, proximal to the ankle.

Electrode position: chest leads

The position of the electrodes for the chest leads is shown in the Figure:
V1: Fourth intercostal space at the right sternal edge.
V2: Fourth intercostal space at the left sternal edge.
V3: Midway between V2 and V4.
V4: Fifth intercostal space in the mid-clavicular line.
V5: Left anterior axillary line at same horizontal level as V4.
V6: Left mid-axillary line at same horizontal level as V4 and V5.

Record

Record a 12-lead ECG at 25 mm/sec with a gain setting of 10 mm/mV. Ensure the printed 12-lead ECG has all the correct details. If the ECG recording is technically correct and of good quality, then the leads and electrodes may be removed from the patient.

Definitions

Artefact: Interference that may impact accurate ECG interpretation, including muscle tremor, wandering baseline, poor electrode contact, patient movement and limb lead reversal.

Electrocardiography: A recording of differences in action potential between sites on the body surface which vary during the cardiac cycle, reflecting differences in voltages within myocardial cells occurring during depolarization and repolarization within each cardiac cycle.

Gain: Size of the ECG trace.

Volt: A measure of electric potential at any point.

Key points
- Ensure correct patient identification details are entered into ECG machine prior to recording ECG.
- Encourage the infant or child to lie as still as possible during the recording.

52 3-lead electrocardiography

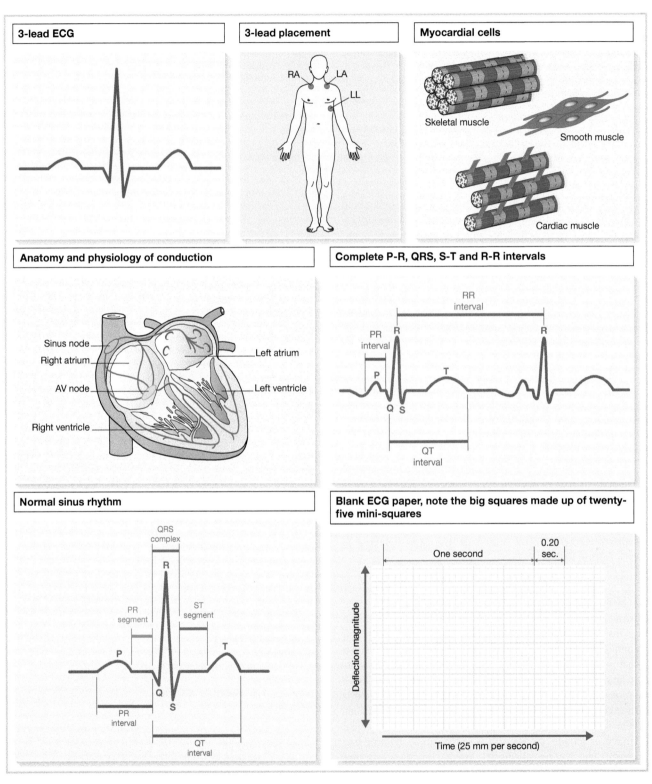

3-lead ECG

3-lead placement

RA   LA

LL

Myocardial cells

Skeletal muscle

Smooth muscle

Cardiac muscle

Anatomy and physiology of conduction

Sinus node
Right atrium
AV node
Right ventricle
Left atrium
Left ventricle

Complete P-R, QRS, S-T and R-R intervals

RR
interval

PR
interval

R   R

P   T

Q S

QT
interval

Normal sinus rhythm

QRS
complex

R

PR
segment

ST
segment

P   T

Q

S

PR
interval

QT
interval

Blank ECG paper, note the big squares made up of twenty-five mini-squares

0.20
sec.

One second

Deflection magnitude

Time (25 mm per second)

Children and Young People's Nursing Skills at a Glance, First Edition. Edited by Elizabeth Gormley-Fleming and Deborah Martin.
© 2018 John Wiley & Sons, Ltd. Published 2018 by John Wiley & Sons, Ltd.

3-lead electrocardiography overview

ECG monitoring looks at the electrical impulses in the cardiac muscle (myocardium). This is generated through placing three electrodes in designated positions. Myocardial cells are striated like skeletal muscles, the action of myocardial cells differs in that movement is involuntary like a smooth muscle and each cell communicates via a 'calcium channel'. This communication causes a contraction or relaxation via a slide-like mechanism. This intrinsic function is controlled by the autonomic nervous system and is influenced by some hormones, including adrenaline and thyroxine. The myocardial cells contract in response to this electrical activity, therefore, having an understanding of what the electrical activity is helps us to understand what the heart is doing and informs a fuller assessment of the infant or child. Electrical impulses, when measured this way, create deviations upwards or downwards from the isoelectric (flat) line. These 'deviations' help us map out the electrical activity and by understanding what normal looks like, we can then identify abnormal electrical impulses. This summary will gave an overview of basic, normal electrocardiology. One heart beat is generally represented by a collection of letters, P, QRS, T and U (rarely recognized). By understanding the normal, the abnormal becomes easier to follow, therefore only the 'normal' will be discussed in this chapter.

The conduction system

One single impulse: Conduction begins in the SA, the sinoatrial node, otherwise known as the 'natural pacemaker'. This is found within the wall of the right atrium, near the superior vena cava. The impulse discharges across both atria, resulting in contraction and depolarization of the AV, the atrioventricular node. The AV node is found in the atrial septum (the dividing wall) near the atrioventricular valves. The impulse then passes down the conduction fibres (Bundle of His) which divide into the left and right bundle branches at the top of the intraventricular septum. These branches terminate in complex fibres called Purkinje fibres, forcing the impulse to spread rapidly across the inner surface of the ventricles causing ventricular contraction. The impulse ends as it moves upwards along the ventricular walls.

One complete cycle

One complete cycle passes through the following impulses:
• *P wave*: This represents atrial depolarization or the passage of electricity from the SA node to both atria. The normal P wave in children and infants is 0.04–0.07 seconds, it is slightly longer in adults.
• *P-R interval*: This is the interval from the beginning of the P wave to the beginning of the QRS complex or the time taken from atrial depolarization to ventricular depolarization. This is usually flat due to a brief delay in conduction. This varies with age and heart rate (HR) – the slower the HR, the longer the P-R interval.
• *QRS complex*: This represents ventricular depolarization or the passage of electricity from the AV node, down the branch bundles in the septum and across both ventricles. The usual length of time for the QRS complex is 0.06–0.08 seconds in infants, 0.1 seconds in children and 0.12 seconds in adolescents.
• *Q-T interval*: This represents the time taken from the beginning of the QRS complex to the end of the T wave. It represents ventricular depolarization and repolarization. The rate is dependent on the age and HR of the patient, the higher the HR, the shorter the Q-T interval.
• *S-T interval*: This represents the interval between the S and T waves and is normally flat, as there is little or no electrical activity at this point.
• *T wave*: This represents ventricular repolarization.

Sinus rhythm

Normal sinus rhythm indicates the beat has arisen from the SA node, represented as a P wave. This P wave is generally of normal shape, length and direction (pointing upwards). This P wave is then followed by a normal P-R interval, then the QRS complex. Every P wave is followed by a QRS and every QRS must be preceded by a P wave for the rhythm to be 'sinus'.

Calculating heart rate using the ECG

While the heart rate is supplied in a variety of forms (manual pulse, on the ECG or Sa02 monitor), calculating the rate is a valuable skill. Using standard ECG recording paper, a useful rough calculation is to divide 300 by the number of large squares between one R-R interval. This is a rough guide but will give an indication of tachycardia or bradycardia. Another method is presuming the standard 12-lead ECG machine is set to record for 10 seconds, multiply the number of QRS complexes in the strip by 6.

Factors that cause significant, life threatening ECG abnormalities

These are the so-called 'reversible causes' and sit within Resuscitation UK's Paediatric Advanced Life Support algorithm (2010). It is worth having an appreciation of the main causes of cardiovascular collapse in children and infants to supplement any attempts to interpret an ECG recording.

Hypoxia: oxygen deprivation causing acidosis.
Hypovolaemia: significant fluid loss, regardless of cause.
Hypo-/hyperkalaemia/metabolic: several electrolytes are crucial for myocardial function, in particular, potassium, calcium and magnesium.
Hypothermia: profound cooling.
Tension pneumothorax: rapid collection of air in the pleural space.
Toxins: these could be ingested medicines or other products,
Tamponade: cardiac tamponade is a collection of fluid (blood, serous fluid or clots) in the pericardial sac, leading to compression of the heart.
Thromboembolism: a blood clot which can migrate.

Key point
• Ensure the correct patient identification details are entered into the ECG machine prior to recording the ECG. This should also include the date and time.

Reference

Resuscitation UK's Paediatric Advanced Life Support algorithm (2015), see https://www.resus.org.uk/resuscitation-guidelines/

53 Pre-operative care and transfer to theatre

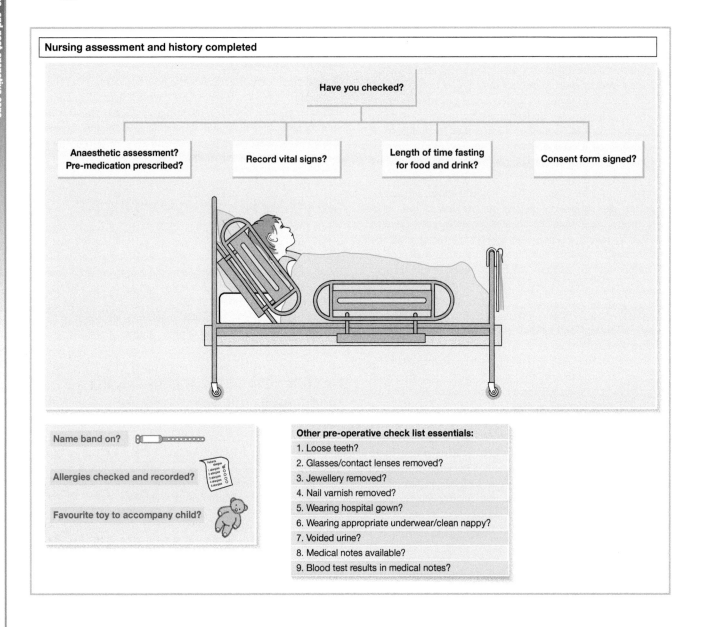

Nursing assessment and history completed

Have you checked?

Anaesthetic assessment?
Pre-medication prescribed?

Record vital signs?

Length of time fasting
for food and drink?

Consent form signed?

Name band on?

Allergies checked and recorded?

Favourite toy to accompany child?

Other pre-operative check list essentials:
1. Loose teeth?
2. Glasses/contact lenses removed?
3. Jewellery removed?
4. Nail varnish removed?
5. Wearing hospital gown?
6. Wearing appropriate underwear/clean nappy?
7. Voided urine?
8. Medical notes available?
9. Blood test results in medical notes?

Children and Young People's Nursing Skills at a Glance, First Edition. Edited by Elizabeth Gormley-Fleming and Deborah Martin.
© 2018 John Wiley & Sons, Ltd. Published 2018 by John Wiley & Sons, Ltd.

Pre-operative care and transfer to theatre overview

It is important to understand the necessity of pre-operative check lists before transferring the child as a patient to the operating theatre. Each point on the check list need to be checked by a number of different professionals, the information recovered from these questions will fully prepare staff for the patient's transfer and during surgery. It is the responsibility of the registered nurse or support worker to complete the theatre check list in full prior to transferring the child to the operating theatre. Once the child's care has been transferred to the theatre staff, a WHO Surgical Safety checklist must be completed. This will allow precautions to be taken or, if necessary, the surgery postponed. The reasons why it is important to follow this check list are listed below. Pre-operative safety checks ensure that the patient is safely prepared for transfer to theatre and for their surgery:

• *Past medical history/previous anaesthetic*: Knowing the child's past medical history will alert staff to any risk factors which could cause problems in surgery, such as breathing problems, heart conditions or previous reactions to anaesthetics. This allows important considerations and preparations to be made to incorporate the patient's conditions or reactions.

• *Pre-operative fasting*: It is important to know the last time the child ate or drank. Fasting must be in accordance with local policy. Normally this fasting period is six hours for food and two hours for clear fluids. The aim of pre-operative fasting is to minimise the volume of the contents of the stomach and thus regurgitation which may lead to aspiration of its contents into the lungs.

• *Known allergies*: A patient's allergy status needs to be clearly recorded so necessary changes can be made in surgery to prevent anaphylaxis during the operation. This may involve changing or avoiding certain medications, or altering equipment being used, e g. latex gloves, depending on the allergy.

• *Baseline observations/weight*: Baseline observations are fundamental in ascertaining the fitness of the patient before surgery. Recording the patient's temperature, pulse and respiration (TPR) and blood pressure (BP) will outline any concerns which can be brought to the attention of the anaesthetist, and will allow comparison for the patient's recovery. Knowing a child's weight is vital for the administration of anaesthetic medication, therefore, before the child is transferred to theatre, a weight needs to be ascertained.

• *Consent form/patient details*: Consent is an important part of medical ethics and is needed before the surgery can take place. It will depend on who is giving consent, if it is the patient's parent only or if the child is competent to give consent as well. The checks should also involving ensuring the person consenting has parental responsibility.

• *ID bracelet/operation site marked*: Before transfer the patient should have an ID bracelet on their wrist. Red or white depending on allergy status, with the correct patient details. This includes the patient's name, date of birth, address, NHS number and hospital number. If required, the patient should have a mark for the operation site before being transferred to theatre. The ID bracelet, the details and operation site will be checked in the anaesthetic room. If any of these is missing, or if the details are incorrect, surgery will be delayed.

• *Seen by anaesthetist/doctor*: Each patient before transfer should be seen by both the anaesthetist and the doctor. They will both go through their necessary check list to ensure the patient is fit for surgery and that they understand the procedure, and the anaesthetic technique which is going to be used. It is at this stage that either the anaesthetist or the doctor may cancel or postpone the surgery if they feel it is not required or it is unsafe to proceed. Therefore, it is paramount that the patient has been seen so that these safety checks can be made before transferring the patient to theatre.

• *Loose teeth*: Loose teeth may be problematic when securing the child's airway during the induction of anaesthesia. Occasionally if very loose they may have to be removed to prevent accidental removal and aspiration into the lungs.

• *Bowels emptied*: Due to the effect of the general anaesthetic, the muscles in the body will relax, therefore, it is best for the patient to have emptied their bowels before going to theatre.

• *Removal of glasses/contact lenses/hearing aids*: The child should be able to wear any visual aids or hearing aids to theatre and these should be removed in the recovery room before surgery. Hearing aids are important as communication with the child is essential at every stage, so they should be removed last.

• *Jewellery/make-up/nail polish removed*: All jewellery should be removed as a safety precaution. If it cannot be removed, adhesive tape should be applied over the item so as it will not catch and pull and cause trauma during surgery. Nail polish should be removed so fingers can be used to position the oxygen saturation monitor probe. Nail polish also harbours microorganism.

• *Pre-medication/medication administered*: The pre-medication should be administered as prescribed. Any additional medication, e.g. inhalers/nebulizers that have been administered prior to transfer to theatre should be noted on the pre-operative check list.

• *Wounds/skin condition*: Wounds and any breaks in the skin/rashes or bruising should be noted on the pre-operative check list.

• *MRSA status*: This should be noted in accordance with local policy.

Key points

• If the child wants to take a familiar toy with them, then this should be permitted.
• The family should be involved in the preparation for theatre.

54 Post-operative recovery

Post-operative recovery

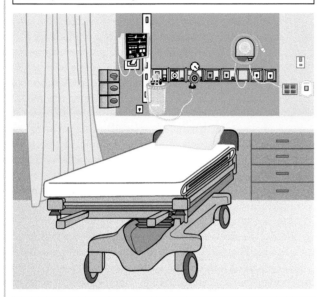

Parent should be invited to the recovery area to sit with their child as soon as possible

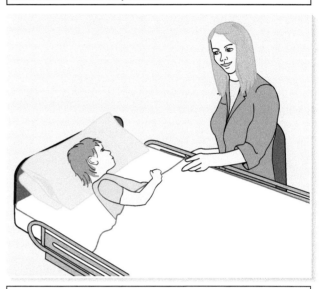

Care in Recovery Unit

Assess:

- Airway
- Breathing
- Cardiovascular status
- Level of consciousness
- Pain
- Temperature
- Post-operative nausea and vomiting
- Wounds
- Drains
- Neurovascular status
- Cannula care

Discharge criteria from Recovery Unit

- Airway patent and breathing normally
- Cardiovascular status normal
- Level of consciousness
- Pain-free
- Normal temperature
- Wounds intact
- No exessive drainage from drains
- No neurovascular compromise (if excessive)

Children and Young People's Nursing Skills at a Glance, First Edition. Edited by Elizabeth Gormley-Fleming and Deborah Martin.
© 2018 John Wiley & Sons, Ltd. Published 2018 by John Wiley & Sons, Ltd.

Post-operative recovery overview

The recovery room provides the patient with a transitioning area between the surgical room and before being transferred back to the ward to begin recovery. The child's recovery period can also be the point where they are at highest risk of developing post-operative complications. Therefore during this transitional period the child will have one-to-one care from a qualified member of staff. The time in which it takes a patient to come around from anaesthetic varies from individual to individual.

Before each child is transferred into recovery, the nursing staff should ensure that the bed space has been checked, and all equipment is accessible and in working order. When the child is transferred from the operating theatre or procedure room to recovery, a detailed handover is provided. This should be given by the anaesthetist, named theatre nurse or, where required, the surgical team, guaranteeing a full detailed account of the patient's operation. Below is a list of details which should be included in the handover to the recovery nurse:

- Patient details.
- Any blood loss/blood products used.
- Known allergies.
- Intravenous fluids given/lines flushed.
- Any medical conditions.
- Post-operative care plan.
- Operative procedure.
- Monitoring required in the recovery room and on return to the ward.
- Any incidents during or before surgery.
- If throat pack has been used and subsequently removed.
- All medication given and required.
- Clear documentation of surgery/medication charts.

Once the child is in the care of the recovery nurse, a full head-to-toe assessment should be carried out. In the assessment the nurse should be focusing on the patient's ABC, airway, breathing and circulation.

- *Airway*: Is the patient self-ventilating, maintaining own airway or needing aided ventilation or airway support? *Observe*: Signs of respiratory distress or airway obstruction.
- *Breathing*: Is the patient's respiratory rate, depth and rhythm within normal range for their age and condition? Work of breathing is normal for the patient. *Observe*: Signs of peripheral and central cyanosis indicated by blue hands, feet, lips, tongue and mucous membranes.
- *Circulation*: Is the patient well perfused, temperature within normal range for patient, capillary refill 2 seconds or less and strength of pulse normal? *Observe*: Continue to monitor clinical presentation of patient's circulation assessment, comparing to normal parameters.

Their neurological status must be checked using AVPU.

A = awake, are they awake?
V = voice, do they respond to your voice?
P = pain, are they in pain?
U = unconscious, are they unconscious?

Other items to be checked are:

- Pain assessment and management are essential components of the immediate post-operative care of the child. Use a pain assessment tool to monitor and document the patient's pain score. If required, administer prescribed analgesia.
- Wounds need to be checked for oozing or active bleeding. It should be noted if the dressings are intact or if they have been replaced.
- Drains need to be monitored for volumes being drained and their insertion sites checked.
- If required, neurovascular status should be checked and recorded.
- Skin integrity should be assessed using a relevant tool.

The child's vital signs should be continuously monitored during their recovery period. This should involve recording the patient's heart rate, respiratory rate, oxygen saturations and blood pressure, ensuring normal parameters are ascertained for the patient's age. Any nausea and vomiting should be recorded and anti-emetics administered. Intravenous infusions should be maintained as prescribed and cannula site checks performed.

Once the child is awake, with a stable airway and cardiovascular system and is pain-free the parents/carers should be asked to come to the recovery area to sit with their child until they are deemed fit for discharge from the recovery unit. The required parameters for discharge from the recovery area are:

- Observations stable and within pre-operative limits.
- Patient is self-ventilating.
- Patient is awake or easily aroused.
- Patient's pain is controlled.
- Nausea/vomiting is absent or controlled.
- All medications have been prescribed.
- Documentation complete/post-operative instructions complete.

A comprehensive handover to the nursing staff is required before the child leaves the recovery area. This handover will need to include the following:

- Patient details.
- Details of procedure.
- How was the child in recovery?
- Any problems that occurred during/after surgery?
- What medication was given and when?
- Record of observations: any vomiting/signs of pain
- Post-operative care plan
- Confirmation of completed documentation.

The nurse collecting the child must be happy that the child's condition is stable. The recovery nurse and the nurse collecting the child should do a top-to-toe assessment of the child together. This is good practice.

Key points

- A systematic assessment is required immediately on arrival into the recovery area.
- All wounds and drains should be assessed and condition noted.
- Ask parents to attend as soon as the child is stable.
- Safe transfer back to the ward is the responsibility of the nurse collecting the child.

55 Basic life support (BLS)

Neutral position

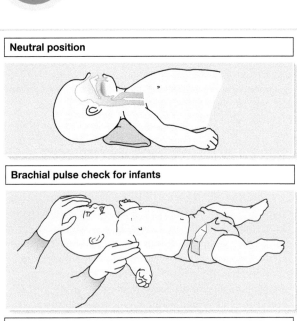

Brachial pulse check for infants

Encircling technique for chest compressions in an infant when performing BLS with two people

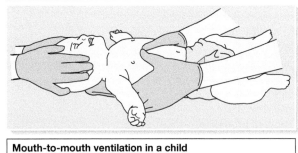

Mouth-to-mouth ventilation in a child

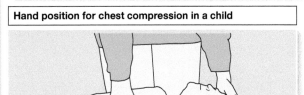

Hand position for chest compression in a child

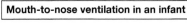

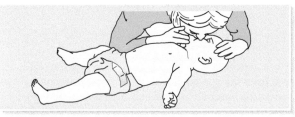

Neutral head position to open airway and two fingers for chest compressions in an infant

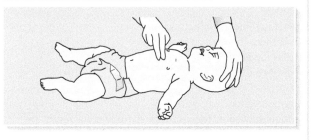

Head tilt chin lift

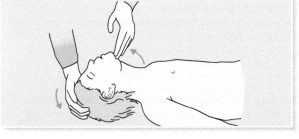

Carotid pulse check for child

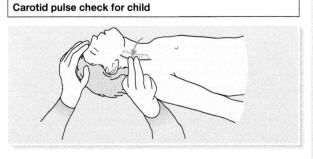

Recovery position for a child

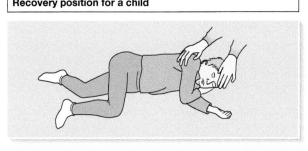

Children and Young People's Nursing Skills at a Glance, First Edition. Edited by Elizabeth Gormley-Fleming and Deborah Martin.
© 2018 John Wiley & Sons, Ltd. Published 2018 by John Wiley & Sons, Ltd.

Basic life support overview

Cardiac arrest in infant and children is less common than in adults. The cause of cardiac arrest in infants and children is secondary to hypoxia. Prompt and effective resuscitation is essential if a successful outcome is to be achieved.

For the purpose of resuscitation, there is a clear delineation between an infant and a child: an infant is aged birth to one year of age; a child is from one year of age to puberty.

Procedure

The safety of the rescuer and the child is paramount.
- Check for responsiveness.
- Gently stimulate the infant or child, ask 'Are you alright?'
- Never shake the infant or child as the cervical spine may be injured.
- If the child does not respond, shout for help.
- Turn the child onto their back and open their airway:
  - neutral position for an infant;
  - modified head tilt chin lift for a child – the sniffing position;
  - head tilt chin lift for an older child.
- Place one hand on the forehead and the other on the bony prominence of the chin. The jaw thrust may be used if there is difficulty opening the airway. To perform a jaw thrust, place your hands on both sides of the child's head, place two or three fingers under the angle of the lower jaw and lift the jaw upwards. This manoeuvre can be used if neck injury is suspected.
- Once the airway is opened, look in the mouth for foreign material. Carefully remove any foreign material that is visible. Do not put fingers into the mouth as they may damage the soft tissues and a blind finger sweep should never be performed.

With the airway open, place your cheek over the infant's or child's mouth, looking towards their feet, and look, listen and feel for 10 seconds:
- Look for chest movement.
- Listen for breathing sounds.
- Feel expired air on your cheek.

If after 10 seconds, the child is not breathing effectively, give five rescue breaths.

Basic life support (BLS) for an infant

- Place mouth over the baby's nose and mouth.
- Deliver each breath over 1 to 1½ seconds and ensure the chest rises and falls.

Basic life support (BLS) for a child

- Place mouth over child's mouth and deliver five breaths of sufficient volume to make the chest rise and fall.
- It is important to take a breath in between delivering each rescue breath.

Circulation check

This should take no more than 10 seconds.
- Look for any signs of life – this may be movements, coughing or return to normal breathing. Agonal breaths or gasping breaths are not normal. Note the child's colour and appearance.
- **For an infant:** locate their brachial pulse and palpate for 10 seconds noting rate and volume. The femoral pulse may also be used. The rate should be 100 or greater. If less than 100 bpm, weak or thready, then chest compressions will need to be commenced.
- The landmark for chest compressions in an infant is one finger's breadth above the xiphisternum.
- Place two fingers (middle and index fingers) on the centre of the chest and give 15 chest compressions. Pressure on the chest should be released between each compression. The chest should be compressed to one third of its depth. The rate of chest compressions will be 100 per minute.
- If two rescuers are present, the second rescuer will deliver chest compression to the infant by encircling the infant's chest with their hands, then with their thumbs side by side, they will compress the centre of the chest while the first rescuer delivers ventilations.
- **For a child:** Check for a pulse by palpating the carotid artery for 10 seconds while also looking for signs of life. If the pulse is less than 60 bpm, then chest compressions will need to be commenced.
- The landmark for chest compressions in a child is two finger breadths above the xiphysternum, then place the heel of one's hand or two hands, one on top of the other, over this area and compress the chest to one third of its depth. Lift the fingers up off the chest to prevent damage to the child's ribs. The rate of chest compressions will be 100 per minute.
- The ratio is 2 breaths and 15 chest compressions for both infant and child. It is important to push hard and fast in order to maintain as adequate a circulation as possible.
- If after one cycle of BLS, help has not arrived, go and get help. It may be possible to carry the infant or child with you and the BLS can be continued.
- The only exception to this is a witnessed cardiac arrest, when BLS would be instigated immediately, then help sought.

Basic life support should be continued until:
- The child recovers, then place in recovery position and check airway and circulation at frequent intervals.
- Help arrives.
- The rescuer becomes exhausted.

Key points
- Early intervention is essential in the chain of survival. The decision to commence BLS should take no longer than 10 seconds.
- Interruptions should be minimized.
- Help must be sought immediately.
- All healthcare professional must have annual updating of BLS skills.

Further reading

Resuscitation Council UK: https://www.resus.org.uk/

56 Advanced resuscitation of the infant and child

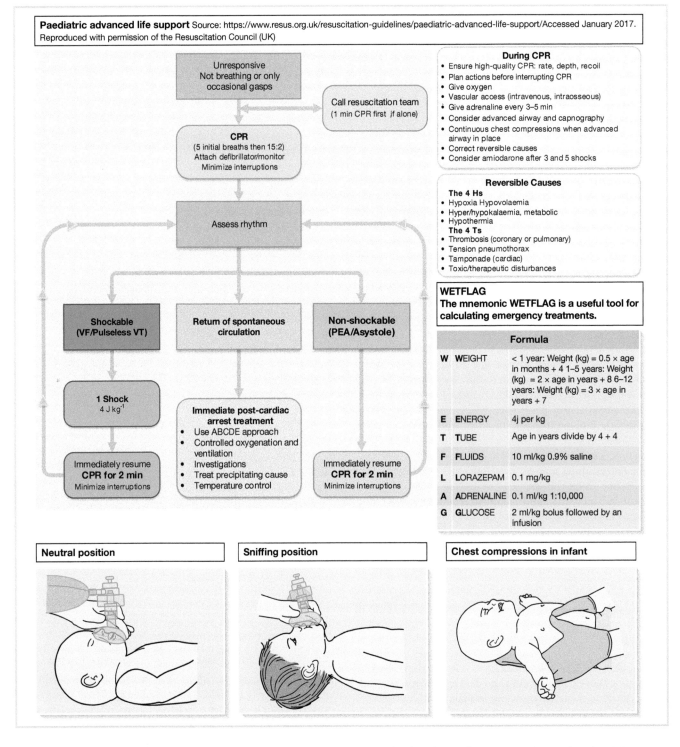

Paediatric advanced life support Source: https://www.resus.org.uk/resuscitation-guidelines/paediatric-advanced-life-support/Accessed January 2017. Reproduced with permission of the Resuscitation Council (UK)

Unresponsive
Not breathing or only occasional gasps

Call resuscitation team
(1 min CPR first if alone)

CPR
(5 initial breaths then 15:2)
Attach defibrillator/monitor
Minimize interruptions

Assess rhythm

Shockable
(VF/Pulseless VT)

Return of spontaneous circulation

Non-shockable
(PEA/Asystole)

1 Shock
4 J kg⁻¹

Immediate post-cardiac arrest treatment
- Use ABCDE approach
- Controlled oxygenation and ventilation
- Investigations
- Treat precipitating cause
- Temperature control

Immediately resume
CPR for 2 min
Minimize interruptions

Immediately resume
CPR for 2 min
Minimize interruptions

During CPR
- Ensure high-quality CPR: rate, depth, recoil
- Plan actions before interrupting CPR
- Give oxygen
- Vascular access (intravenous, intraosseous)
- Give adrenaline every 3–5 min
- Consider advanced airway and capnography
- Continuous chest compressions when advanced airway in place
- Correct reversible causes
- Consider amiodarone after 3 and 5 shocks

Reversible Causes
The 4 Hs
- Hypoxia Hypovolaemia
- Hyper/hypokalaemia, metabolic
- Hypothermia
The 4 Ts
- Thrombosis (coronary or pulmonary)
- Tension pneumothorax
- Tamponade (cardiac)
- Toxic/therapeutic disturbances

WETFLAG
The mnemonic WETFLAG is a useful tool for calculating emergency treatments.

		Formula
W	WEIGHT	< 1 year: Weight (kg) = 0.5 × age in months + 4 1–5 years: Weight (kg) = 2 × age in years + 8 6–12 years: Weight (kg) = 3 × age in years + 7
E	ENERGY	4j per kg
T	TUBE	Age in years divide by 4 + 4
F	FLUIDS	10 ml/kg 0.9% saline
L	LORAZEPAM	0.1 mg/kg
A	ADRENALINE	0.1 ml/kg 1:10,000
G	GLUCOSE	2 ml/kg bolus followed by an infusion

Neutral position

Sniffing position

Chest compressions in infant

Advanced resuscitation of the infant and child overview

Cardiac arrest in infants and children is an uncommon event with the incidence said to be 2.28 per 100,000 person years, with the 0–2 age group accounting for the highest incidence (2.1 per 100,000 person years), dropping to 0.61 in the age group 3–13

years. The data for cardiac arrest in hospital in the UK is somewhat harder to determine.

Definitions

Child – is over 1 year and up to puberty
CPR – cardiopulmonary resuscitation
Infant – is under 12 months

Children and Young People's Nursing Skills at a Glance, First Edition. Edited by Elizabeth Gormley-Fleming and Deborah Martin.
© 2018 John Wiley & Sons, Ltd. Published 2018 by John Wiley & Sons, Ltd.

Neonate – is an infant in the first 28 days of life
Newborn – an infant immediately following delivery
NICU – Neonatal Intensive Care Unit
PICU – paediatric intensive care unit
ROSC – return of spontaneous circulation
SCBU – Special Care Baby Unit.

Newborn life support is not covered in this chapter, however, a baby in the first 28 days of life (outside of the NICU/SCBU/delivery setting) should be treated as an infant in relation to the algorithm to be followed.

Causes of cardiac arrest

Secondary cardiopulmonary arrest is more common in the paediatric patient with causes including:

- sudden infant death syndrome;
- congenital anomalies (more common in the 0–2 age group);
- trauma;
- airway-related events/respiratory illness;
- drowning.

The key factors that determine outcome from paediatric cardiac arrest are:

- witnessed cardiac arrest;
- chain of survival:
  - early recognition and call for help;
  - establishing basic life support (BLS);
  - early defibrillation;
  - post-resuscitation care.

ABCDE assessment

The assessment and intervention for any seriously ill or injured child should follow the ABCDE approach:

A = airway (Ac for airway and cervical spine stabilization for the injured child)
B = breathing
C = circulation (with haemorrhage control in injured child)
D = disability (level of consciousness and neurological status)
E = exposure to allow full examination (while respecting dignity and temperature conservation)

The sequence of actions can be found in the paediatric advanced life support algorithm and includes:

- Use ABCDE approach to assessment.
- Recognition of cardiac arrest and call for the appropriate team.
- Establish BLS.
- Oxygenate:
  - Place the infant in the neutral position.
  - Place the child in the sniffing position.
  - Use 100% oxygen in the infant and child until ROSC.
- Ventilate:
  - Use a self-inflating bag device.
  - Give five rescue breaths.
  - Observe for adequate chest movement.
  - Consider airway adjuncts such as the oropharyngeal airway or laryngeal mask airway (LMA).
- Start chest compressions:
  - ratio of 15:2;
  - rate of at least 100 but not greater than 120 per minute;
  - depth of compression at least 1/3 of the AP diameter.
- Attach a defibrillator and assess rhythm:
  - Consider front and back pads in the infant.
  - Use paediatric pads in the 1–8 year group.
  - Use adult pads in the > 8 year group.
- Treat non-shockable rhythm with continuous CPR and adrenaline.

- Treat shockable rhythm with defibrillator and continue CPR.
- Consider reversible causes throughout the cardiac arrest.

Reversible causes

The reversible causes of cardiac arrest are described as the 4 H's and the 4 T's. These reversible causes should be considered in all cardiac arrest situations. The order of the reversible causes in the figure does not correspond to the incidence of the reversible cause. The most likely reversible cause will be different in each cardiac arrest and will be determined by the clinician using the history of events and clinical presentation as a guide.

Parents

Parental presence during cardiopulmonary resuscitation has been much debated. It is evident from research that parents often want to remain present and staff often feel this is appropriate. However, in order for this to be successful, you must be able to ensure a dedicated nurse is available to support the parent(s) throughout the resuscitation attempt.

Human factors

Although knowledge and skill in advanced resuscitation techniques are considered the most important factor in treating the patient in cardiac arrest, human factors (the discipline concerned with understanding relationships and human interaction) may also play a part in achieving positive outcomes. The human factor principles that may specifically be addressed include leadership, team work, situational awareness and communication. Teams that have good leadership in particular have been found in simulated cardiac arrest to be more successful. Human factors training is slowly being incorporated into medicine and nursing training and may in future be incorporated into advance life support training.

Outcomes from cardiac arrest

A positive outcome from an out-of-hospital cardiac arrest in this group of patients is higher than that of the adult population. One study in 2013 reported an 18.5% survival to discharge rate with 92% of survivors still alive at 1 year, whereas a study in 2012 reports a 32% survival rate. The data from these studies was further analysed and witnessed arrest with shockable rhythm further improved outcome as well as shorter duration of cardiac arrest and ROSC prior to arrival in hospital.

Data from in hospital cardiac arrest reports increased survival of up to 48% with 76% of those surviving with a good neurological outcome.

Post-cardiac arrest care

Following ROSC, pulse oximetry should be used and oxygen should be titrated to achieve saturation levels of 94–98%. The airway should be stabilized and the child transferred to the paediatric intensive care unit (PICU) area for ongoing stabilization and care.

In the adolescent who remains comatose following cardiac arrest, therapeutic hypothermia for 24 hours may be beneficial. Evidence is still emerging, however, it may also be considered in the child.

Key points

- Recognition of the sick child and prompt intervention are key to a successful outcome.
- Organization and team work are important in managing the child in cardiac arrest.
- Provide a nurse to care for the parents if they are present in the resuscitation room.

57 # Transfer of the critically ill child

Transportation medication chart

CHILDREN'S ACUTE TRANSPORT SERVICE
ELECTRONIC DRUG CHART FOR REFERRING HOSPITALS

PATIENT NAME & HOSPITAL NO. (or addressograph label)	ALLERGIES/SENSITIVITIES	DATE OF BIRTH	WEIGHT (IN KG)		CALCULATE
	NAME & POSITION OF PERSON RECORDING ALLERGIES	DATE OF CHART 19/11/2014	DATE WEIGHED		PRINT RESET

Allergies must be documented before prescribing/administration except in exceptional circumstances

DRUG		PUT	IN	DILUENT (circle as appropriate)	RATE RANGE			EQUIVALENT TO DOSE RANGE	PRESCRIBER SIGNATURE	TIME MADE	NURSE'S SIGNATURE
ANALGESICS, SEDATIVES AND MUSCLE RELAXANTS											
MORPHINE		mg	50 ml			to	ml/hr	10–40 microgram/kg/hr			
MIDAZOLAM		mg	50 ml			to	ml/hr				
*VECURONIUM		mg	25 ml			to	ml/hr	1–4 microgram/kg/min			
*ATRACURIUM		mg	50 ml			to	ml/hr				
* FENTANYL		mg	50 ml			to	ml/hr	2–8 microgram/kg/hr			
KETAMINE		mg	50 ml			to	ml/hr	10–40 microgram/kg/min			
VASOACTIVE AGENTS											
ADRENALINE		mg	50 ml			to	ml/hr	0.1–0.5 microgram/kg/min			
NORADRENALINE		mg	50 ml			to	ml/hr	0.1–0.5 microgram/kg/min			
DOPAMINE											
Central line		mg	50 ml			to	ml/hr	5–20 microgram/kg/min			
Peripheral line		mg	50 ml			to	ml/hr	5–20 microgram/kg/min			
DOBUTAMINE		mg	50 ml			to	ml/hr	5–20 microgram/kg/min			
DUCT PATENCY											
ALPROSTADIL		mg	50 ml			to	ml/hr	10–100 nanogram/kg/min			
DINOPROSTONE		mg	50 ml			to	ml/hr	5–50 nanogram/kg/min			
INTRAVENOUS BRONCHODILATORS											
SALBUTAMOL		mg	50 ml			to	ml/hr	1–2 microgram/kg/min			
*AMINOPHYLLINE											
Age 1 mon-12 yrs	250	mg	50 ml			to	ml/hr	1 mg/kg/hr			
Age 12 yrs-18 yrs	250	mg	50 ml			to	ml/hr	0.5–0.7 mg/kg/hr			

* If patient is obese, adjust doses for ideal body weight

Baby prepared for transfer

Peripherally inserted central catheter (PICC)
Endotracheal tube
Pulse oximeter Also one on left foot
Chest tube
Temperature monitor
EKG probes
Nasogastric tube
Umbilical arterial catheter

Trolley with portable equipment for transfer

Infusion pump
Monitor
Fluids
Endotracheal tube
Transport mechanical ventilator
Transport bed

Children and Young People's Nursing Skills at a Glance, First Edition. Edited by Elizabeth Gormley-Fleming and Deborah Martin.
© 2018 John Wiley & Sons, Ltd. Published 2018 by John Wiley & Sons, Ltd.

Transfer of the critically ill child overview

Every paediatric emergency department should provide all the essential steps that are needed for a child. This should include initial assessment, resuscitation, stabilization and transport of the critically or injured child. Most critically ill children will first receive initial hospital care in their local emergency department for stabilization, then will be transferred to their nearest tertiary centre, depending on the availability of a bed.

Stabilization

A critically ill child will mostly present at a local district hospital. During a resuscitation there should be a paediatric registrar or consultant leading the team during the CPR and when stabilizing the child. Other team members include an anaesthetist consultant, paediatric junior doctor and a paediatric nurse. If the child is deteriorating, the next stage is preparation for intubation and ventilation. The nursing team will then prepare all the drugs needed for the retrieval team. The child will be retrieved by a team of specialist nurses and doctors. The Children's Acute Transport Service (CATS) retrieval team complete the electronic drug chart (see Transportation medication chart) as a quick tool for referring a child. By adding the weight and date of birth of the child it will automatically calculate the doses and then be ready to print to use as a drug chart.

Intubation/ventilation equipment and monitoring

Intubation is required when the child has difficulty in maintaining their own airway, is in respiratory failure, to minimise oxygen consumption and to maximise oxygen delivery and to prevent secondary brain injury. It is important to intubate the child for a number of reasons; the patient's airway is protected and secured, to provide positive pressure ventilation to children with respiratory failure or serious hypoxaemia, and to support the respiratory function during anaesthesia. A systematic approach to the management of the critically ill child is essential to ensure the required interventions can be delivered.

Airway

Endotracheal (ET) tubes will be used to maintain the airway; they can be cuffed or uncuffed, this will depend on the age of the child. Ensure a secured airway by good positioning of the child's airway and with no significant leak from the ET tube. Add positive end expiratory pressure (PEEP) as soon as possible to the ventilation circuit. The gastric tube is also used to allow free drainage from the stomach in the ventilated child. Always discuss with the consultant of the transfer service about the induction agent and prepare the fluid bolus and possible dopamine infusion. A chest X-ray post intubation will be needed with a copy for the transport team.

Breathing

Ensure adequate ventilation by monitoring end tidal carbon dioxide ($ETCO_2$). If there are ventilation problems, it is essential to rule out any ET tube-related problems urgently. These may include inadequate sedation or paralysis, large leak around the ET tube in a child who requires high ventilatory pressures. The anaesthetist will need to reassess the child and review intubation. Suctioning and physiotherapy will be considered if there is an unintended endobronchial intubation which may result in a tension pneumothorax, which must be drained. All the ventilation strategies must be discussed with the transfer consultant. There must be appropriate targets for blood gases, all depending on the clinical condition of the child.

Circulation

In a life-threatening situation, two good intravenous access points are a priority. A peripheral or interosseous (IO) inotrope infusion can be used until there is a central access. The blood gases can be taken from a peripheral line until the arterial line is placed. Continuous blood pressure (BP) readings must be taken until the placement of the arterial line. Circulatory support can be discussed with the transfer consultant for the most appropriate inotrope. Early aggressive fluid resuscitation and inotropes may be required. In the circulation stage, you need to check $ETCO_2$ tracing to monitor any poor cardiac output and frequent BP checks until the arterial line is placed.

Disability

See chart to commence adequate sedation and paralysis of the child. Monitoring of blood glucose levels is essential along with pupil reactions and body temperature. To control temperature, a bear hugger may be used if the child is hypothermic and aim for normothermia, unless cooling is indicated. Maintaining fluids and consideration of a urinary catheter are important to monitor the output of the child or avoid fluid retention. Further tests such as CT scan or a blood film may be requested by the transfer consultant, and antibiotic infusions may be considered. Once the child is stable, all the notes must be photocopied and X-rays sent must be ready for the retrieval team.

Family

Care of the family is important and they need to be prepared for the transportation of their child. It is not always possible for the parents to be able to accompany the child so arrangements need to be made for the parents to travel to the receiving hospital. They may not be in a fit state to drive and this should be considered. Careful documentation of discussion with the family about their child's condition should occur.

Key points

- Early contact with the retrieval team is essential.
- Communicate with the family and details of the retrieval need to be shared with them.

58 Phototherapy

Conventional phototherapy

Fibre optic phototherapy

A sample of bilirubin thresholds for phototherapy and exchange transfusion in babies with hyperbilirubinaemia

Baby's name _____

Hospital number _____   Time of birth _____

Date of birth _____   **26** weeks gestation

Direct antiglobulin test _____

Multiple
Single

Shade for phototherapy

Total serum bilirubin (micromol/litre)

550
500
450
400
350
300
250
200
150
100
50
0

Exchange transfusion

Phototherapy

0 1 2 3 4 5 6 7 8 9 10 11 12 13 14

Days from birth

Baby's blood group _____   Mother's blood group _____

Children and Young People's Nursing Skills at a Glance, First Edition. Edited by Elizabeth Gormley-Fleming and Deborah Martin.
© 2018 John Wiley & Sons, Ltd. Published 2018 by John Wiley & Sons, Ltd.

Phototherapy overview

Jaundice is one of the most common conditions in newborn babies needing medical attention. Jaundice refers to the yellow colour of the skin and the whites of the eyes caused by excess bilirubin in the blood, also known as hyperbilirubinaemia. Bilirubin is produced by the normal breakdown of red blood cells and is excreted as bile through the intestine. Jaundice occurs when bilirubin builds up faster than a newborn's liver can break it down and pass it from the body. Jaundice can affect both term and pre-term newborns, however, the pre-term infants are at higher risk due to the pre-maturity of their organs, especially the liver. In most babies, jaundice is harmless, however, if the bilirubin is unconjugated (bilirubin which is not water-soluble, hence not excreted in the urine), then using phototherapy can be beneficial in treating these infants.

What is phototherapy?

Phototherapy refers to treatment with light. The equipment consists of a number of fluorescent light tubes which emit light in the blue-green band of the visible spectrum (425–475 nm). The blue-green light converts the unconjugated bilirubin to a harmless isomer which can easily be excreted in water.

Types of phototherapy

• *Conventional phototherapy*: Phototherapy given using a single light source (not fibre optic) that is positioned above the baby.
• *Fibre optic phototherapy*: Phototherapy given using a single light source that comprises a light generator, a fibre optic cable through which the light is carried and a flexible light pad, on which the baby is placed or that is wrapped around the baby.

Equipment

• Appropriate light source: overhead lamps/fibre optic light source is bilisoft.
• Eye-shield: with appropriate size to suit the pre-term/term infants.
• Tape measure: to adjust the distance of the light from the infant as per manufacturer's guidelines.
• Appropriate phototherapy charts for the gestation of the infant (refer to NICE treatment threshold graphs). Check the bilirubin levels and plot them on the correct chart.
Ensure all phototherapy equipment is maintained and used according to the manufacturer's guidelines.

Procedure

• Explain the need for phototherapy to parents and obtain consent. Additional information can be supplied with information leaflets.
• Wash hands.
• Remove all of the baby's clothing except for the nappy.
• The baby should wear the smallest appropriate nappy to maximize skin exposure.
• Remove any lotions or creams applied to the baby as this will cause the treatment to be ineffective and create skin irritation.
• If possible, cleanse the skin with warm water prior to the procedure to ensure good skin integrity is maintained and the treatment is effective.
• Apply the eye-shield prior to commencing the light.

• If the overhead light is used, then adjust the distance as per manufacturer's instruction and turn the lights on.
• Check the body temperature prior to the treatment and monitor the baby's temperature three-hourly and ensure the baby is kept in a thermo-neutral environment (36.8–37.2°C).
• Ensure the infant has good fluid intake. Monitor hydration by daily weighing of the baby and assessing wet nappies.
• Change position with nappy care to obtain effective phototherapy to cover whole body.
• Monitor bilirubin regularly.
• Document time of commencement and completion of phototherapy in the neonate's health care records and on the phototherapy chart.
• Support parents and carers and encourage them to interact with the baby.
• When serum bilirubin is 50 micromol/litre below the threshold, stop the phototherapy.
• Check serum bilirubin for rebound 12–18 hours after ceasing phototherapy.

Potential hazards disadvantages

Hypo/hyperthermia: The infants who are nursed in a cot have a high risk of developing hypothermia (low temperature). Bilisoft (fibre optic) pads can be a solution to this as the infant can be further wrapped with a blanket. An incubator would be better for ideal phototherapy as it can ensure light and thermoregulation.
• *Risk of eye damage*: Radiation from the phototherapy light can cause retinal damage, hence eye protection with the eye-shield is necessary. This should be checked at least every 4–6 hours to check for any corneal skin breakdown. Also ensure that the eye-shields do not occlude the nares as this can interfere with breathing.
• *Insensible loss/dehydration*: Phototherapy may decrease the bowel transit time and result in diarrhoea, probably as a result of bowel wall irritation caused by the presence of photo-isomers of bilirubin. Jaundiced infants are commonly drowsy and may not wake up for feeds. An increase in the fluid requirement of 10–25% may be considered.
• *Skin irritation and damage*: Deposits of bile salts in the skin can cause irritation and itching. Redness and inflammation can occur from a photosensitive reaction. Avoid using lotions and creams, inspect the skin regularly, and a position change is recommended.
• *Parental anxiety and separation from the baby*: Parents are in a vulnerable state usually post-natally and the infant having jaundice and phototherapy with eye coverage can upset them. If possible, nurse the infant with the mother in a post-natal ward.

Key points
• Eyes must be protected.
• The baby's temperature should be recorded and maintained within normal range as hypo/hyperthermia may occur.
• Fluids need to be increased by 10–25%.

Further reading

National Institute for Health and Care Excellence (2010) Jaundice in newborn babies under 28 days. NICE clinical guidance CG98. Available at: https://www.nice.org.uk/Guidance/CG98

59 Care of the umbilicus

Newborn baby with unclamped cord
Source: By Ernest F (Own work) [GFDL(http://www.gnu.org/copyleft/fdl.html) or CC-BY-SA-3.0(http://creativecommons.org/licenses/by-sa/3.0/)], via Wikimedia Commons

Newborn baby with unclamped cord
Source: https://commons.wikimedia.org/wiki/File:Umbilicalcord.jpg?uselang=en-gb

Cord stump on day 1 showing vessels

Cord stump on day 2

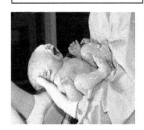
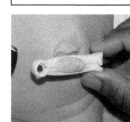
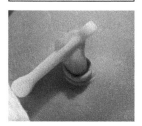

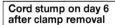
OPEN CORD CARE

Cord drying out day 4

Cord stump on day 6 after clamp removal

Cord stump healing after clamp removal
Source: https://commons.wikimedia.org/wiki/File:Umbilicalstump.jpg?uselang=en-gb

The umbilical stump after stump separation

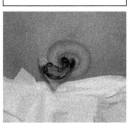
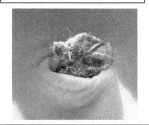
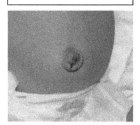

Observation of the cord

- Observe the umbilicus and surrounding area for signs of bleeding and infection.
- Look for inflammation/swelling/pus/offensive odour from the cord.
- Note any abnormality, e.g. granuloma, hernia/a red flare around the cord stump (erythema)/pyrexia.
- Signs of lethargy and poor feeding alongside the signs of infection point to systemic involvement. Complications of the above include septicaemia and peritonitis. Broad-spectrum antibiotic cover is the treatment of choice.
- If a microbiology swab result is available, specific antibiotics can be targeted.
- The prevalence of a moist or sticky cord base is not necessarily a positive sign of infection.
- If the baby is alert, feeding well and afebrile, then the chances of infection remain low.
- Observation is the only treatment required in this instance.

Cleaning the umbilical area (if there are signs of infection)

- Co-ordinate procedure to minimize handling the baby. Prepare the baby, lie the baby supine, remove the nappy but keep the baby warm.
- Collect equipment: clean nappy, plain water and gauze, bacterial swab and request form for microbiology, appropriate protective equipment, including apron and gloves.
- Standard precautions. Wash hands immediately prior to handling baby.
- To clean the umbilicus:
    - Pour water onto an open gauze pack and gently wipe from clean to dirty area.
    - Using a dry clean gauze, pat the cord area dry – do not rub or pull at the stump, any residue which remains should be left to fall off in time.
    - Involve the parents/carers in re-applying the nappy and making the baby comfortable.
- Dispose of used equipment according to the waste management policy and perform a hand wash.

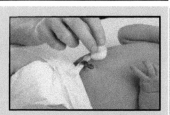

Umbilical cord: Source: https://commons.wikimedia.org/wiki/File:Umbilicalcord.jpg?uselang=en-gb

Children and Young People's Nursing Skills at a Glance, First Edition. Edited by Elizabeth Gormley-Fleming and Deborah Martin.
© 2018 John Wiley & Sons, Ltd. Published 2018 by John Wiley & Sons, Ltd.

Care of the umbilicus overview

During pregnancy, the umbilical cord connects the placenta to the growing foetus and serves to provide nutrients and oxygen for growth while removing metabolic waste products and carbon dioxide simultaneously. The cord consists of two arteries and one vein covered by a mucoid connective tissue known as Wharton's jelly, enclosed by a thin layer of mucous membrane, a continuation of the amnion. The Wharton's jelly gives the cord a translucent appearance but it can be stained green due to meconium or yellow if the newborn baby has early hyperbilirubinaemia (jaundice).

Following delivery, the cord quickly starts to dry out, harden and turns necrotic (dry gangrene) assisted by exposure to the air. Separation of the umbilical cord continues at the junction of the cord and the skin of the abdomen, with leucocyte infiltration and subsequent digestion of the cord. During this normal process, small amounts of cloudy mucoid material may collect at the junction. This may wrongly be interpreted as pus. A moist and/ or sticky cord may present, but this too is part of the normal physiological process.

The umbilical vessels remain patent for several days, so the risk of infection remains high until separation. Colonization of the area begins within hours of birth because of non-pathogenic organisms such as *Staphylococci* and *Diphtheroid* bacilli passing from mother to baby via skin contact. Immediate skin-to-skin contact following delivery is important because it will encourage non-pathogenic colonization from mother to baby. It is also known to encourage bonding, attachment and successful breastfeeding.

Pathogenic or harmful bacteria, however, such as *Coliforms* and *Streptococci* can be spread by poor hygiene, poor handwashing techniques and especially by cross-infection, and can track up the umbilical stump causing infection.

Care at birth

At birth, the baby is still attached to the mother via the umbilical cord and then is separated from the placenta by clamping the cord. This clamping is one part of the third stage of labour (the time from birth of the baby until delivery of the placenta) and the timing can vary according to clinical policy and practice. For many years now, standard care during the delivery of the placenta has been to clamp the cord immediately at birth. However, it is more commonplace now in well newborn babies that a delay in clamping is carried out for at least 30 seconds to enable the baby to obtain extra blood volume in order to raise early haemoglobin concentrations, to prevent anaemia and increase the iron stores in the neonatal period.

Following clamping, the cord is cut to leave a stump. The cord and the placenta are then examined to ensure it contains two arteries and one vein. From birth for the first few days, the umbilical vessels are still patent and may be cannulated for arterial or venous access to allow administration of drugs and intravenous fluids, invasive blood pressure monitoring, blood sampling and exchange transfusion. The associated risks of cannulation include obstructed blood flow to major vessels, potentially causing ischaemia to a lower limbs, infection and thrombosis.

Care after birth

The cord usually separates between five and 15 days after birth. The figure shows the cord drying out in stages from day 2, to day 4, after clamp removal on day 6 and finally once the cord stump has separated leaving a clean, dry umbilicus.

Open cord care comprises the following:
• Leave the cord open to the air to allow the cord to dry out naturally.
• Minimal handling of the cord and surrounding area to cut down the risk of cross-infection.
• Clothes should be clean and loose fitting to allow air to circulate.
• Fold down the nappy so that the cord is left exposed.

However, the umbilical cord and surrounding area are a potential source of post-natal complication for a newborn baby, requiring regular observation and care until separation occurs. It is therefore essential to keep the cord clean and dry to prevent infection using clean water only to clean if necessary. The use of various baby products, alcohol wipes, dyes, creams and powders have been used in the past but have only served to increase infection rates of the umbilicus. Generally, it is now accepted that the more the cord is treated, the longer it will take to separate as products delay the natural healing process. Prolonged cord separation rates are associated with an increased risk of infection.

Finally, cord care is an ideal area to involve the parents and teach them the fundamental hygiene needs of their baby. Respect for cultural beliefs and traditions is vital in the cutting and cleaning of the umbilicus. Parents should be informed at all times that the cord needs to be closely observed, the reasons why and advised on how they should keep the cord clean and dry, along with other important areas of parent craft.

Key points
• Umbilical cord care focuses on keeping the stump clean, dry and free of infection.
• Leave the umbilical cord open to the air or cover with clean, loose clothing during the time from birth to stump separation.
• Leave the stump alone unless it looks or becomes infected, contaminated by faeces or urine. Clean, if necessary, with plain water only.
• Observe the umbilicus and surrounding area for bleeding and signs of infection as the umbilical area is a potential source of colonization by pathogenic bacteria.

Further reading

McDonald, S.J., Middleton, P., Dowswell, T. and Morris, P.S. (2013) Effect of timing of umbilical cord clamping of term infants on maternal and neonatal outcomes. *Cochrane Database of Systematic Reviews*. Issue 7. Art. No.: CD004074.

National Institute for Health and Care Excellence (2006) Postnatal care: routine postnatal care of women and their babies. NICE clinical guidance CG37. Available at: http://www.nice .org.uk/guidance/cg37/resources/guidance-postnatal-care-pdf (accessed 18 February 2015).

Rabe, H., Diaz-Rossello, J.L., Duley, L. and Dowswell, T. (2012) Effect of timing of umbilical cord clamping and other strategies to influence placental transfusion at preterm birth on maternal and infant outcomes. *Cochrane Database of Systematic Reviews*. Issue 8. Art. No.:CD003248.

Zupan, J., Garner, P., and Omari, A.A.A. (2004) Topical umbilical cord care at birth. *Cochrane Database of Systematic Reviews*. Issue 3. Art. No.: CD001057. DOI:10.1002/14651858. CD001057.pub2.

60 Hand washing

Hand-washing technique

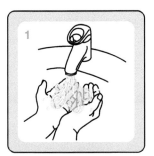

Wet hand with water

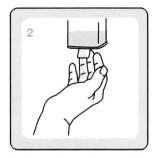

Apply enough soap to cover all hand surfaces

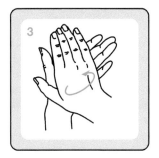

Rub hands palm to palm

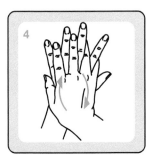

Right palm over left dorsum with interlaced fingers and vice versa

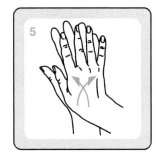

Palm to palm with fingers interlaced

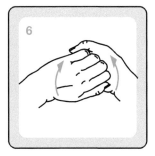

Backs of fingers to opposing palms with fingers interlocked

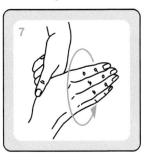

Rotational rubbing of left thumb clasped in right palm and vice versa

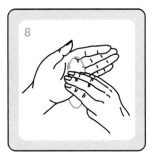

Rotational rubbing, backwards and forwards with clasped fingers of right hand in left palm and vice versa

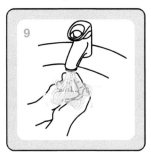

Rinse hands with water

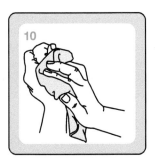

Dry thoroughly with a single use towel

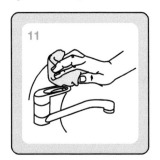

Use towel to turn off tap

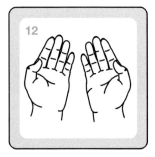

...and your hands are safe

Children and Young People's Nursing Skills at a Glance, First Edition. Edited by Elizabeth Gormley-Fleming and Deborah Martin.
© 2018 John Wiley & Sons, Ltd. Published 2018 by John Wiley & Sons, Ltd.

Hand-washing overview

Hand hygiene is the single most important factor in reducing hospital-acquired infections (HAI). Hands are a major source of the transmission of organisms since they are point of contact during patient care. Hand hygiene is the decontamination via the use of hand rub – using an alcohol-based formula – or hand washing with soap and water, in order to reduce the number of bacteria on the hands. Health care-associated infections are of concern to all and good hand hygiene is vital in order to avoid the transmission of organisms to vulnerable neonates, infants and children.

Dangers of not carrying out hand hygiene

Without the process of hand hygiene or if there is insufficient hand hygiene, there is a higher risk of the transmission of bacteria. Unclean hands can do the following:

* Transfer the patient's own microorganisms into germ-free areas of the patient's own body while carrying out their care or treatment.
* Transfer microorganisms from one patient to another patient.
* Transfer microorganisms from the environment and equipment to a patient.
* Catch microorganisms from contact with patients, the environment or equipment, which place health care staff at risk of infection.

Methicillin-resistant *Staphylococcus aureus* (MRSA) and *Clostridium difficile* (C. difficile) are two of the most common type of HAIs.

Carrying out hand hygiene

Nails should be kept short and free from nail varnish. Artificial nails are not permitted. Hospital policy should be followed in relation to the wearing of rings. Wrist watches should not be worn.

Hand rubbing (duration 20–30 seconds)

It is most beneficial to patient safety to place hand rub dispensers at the point of care, that is, the patient's immediate environment where health care staff-to-patient contact or treatment takes place. Safety must be considered in children's wards, so hand rub dispensers should not be accessible to young children. An alcohol-based formulation is the preferred routine for hand antisepsis if hands are not visibly soiled.

Apply the product from the dispenser. Follow hand hygiene movements steps 1–8. Allow hands to dry.

Hand washing (duration 40–60 seconds)

An effective hand-washing technique consists of three stages: preparation, washing and rinsing, and drying. Use the hand-washing method via using soap and water when hands are visibly dirty or visibly soiled with blood or other body fluids.

* Wet hands thoroughly under running tepid water.
* Dispense one dose of soap into cupped hands.
* Follow hand hygiene movements steps 1–12 as in Figure.
* After, rinse hands with warm water and dry thoroughly with paper towel. Cloth towels must NOT be used to avoid cross-contamination.
* Turn off the taps using a 'hands-free' technique; using your elbows is an example. Where this is not possible, the paper towel used to dry the hands can be used to turn off the tap to avoid re-contaminating hands. Finally, dispose of the paper towel without re-contaminating hands.

Hand hygiene movement steps

The step-by-step technique must be followed if hands are to be decontaminated effectively.

1 Turn on taps and let water run until temperature is comfortable.
2 Wet hands up to wrists.
3 Apply soap.
4 Rub hands palm to palm.
5 Right palm over the back of the other hand with interlaced fingers and vice versa.
6 Palm to palm with fingers interlaced.
7 Back of fingers to opposing palms with fingers interlocked.
8 Rotational rubbing of left thumb clasped in right palm and vice versa.
9 Rotational rubbing, backwards and forwards with clasped fingers of right hand in left palm and vice versa.
10 Rinse off soap.
11 Turn off taps with elbows or paper towel.
12 Dry hands and wrists thoroughly with disposable paper towel.
13 Dispose of paper towel as per local policy. Bin should be foot-operated.
14 Social hand washing normally takes 10–15 seconds.

The five moments of carrying out hand hygiene

There are five crucial moments in patient care when hand hygiene is used. These should be carried out regardless of whether gloves are used or not:

1 *Before patient contact.* To protect the patient against harmful germs carried on your hands.
2 *Before clean/aseptic task.* To protect the patient against harmful germs, including the patient's own, from entering his/her body.
3 *After body fluid exposure risk.* To protect yourself and the health care environment from harmful patient germs.
4 *After patient contact.* To protect yourself and the health care environment from harmful patient germs.
5 *After contact with patient's surroundings.* To protect yourself and the health care environment from harmful patient germs.

Hand care

Health care staff need to maintain healthy skin on their hands. Employers should manage the risks of work-related contact dermatitis arising from hand hygiene measures. Regular use of a protective hand cream or lotion is essential. After hand rubbing or hand washing, let your hands dry completely before putting on gloves. If a particular soap, hand wash or alcohol-based product causes skin irritation, an occupational health team should be consulted.

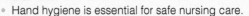

Key points

* Hand hygiene is essential for safe nursing care.
* Nails should be kept short.
* Local policy should be adhered to in regard to the wearing of rings.

61 Aseptic non-touch technique

Hand-washing steps: see Chapter 60

Key parts of equipment

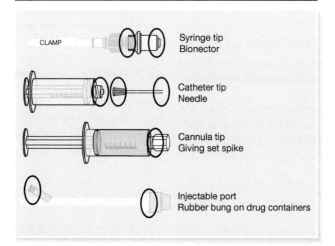

CLAMP

Syringe tip
Bionector

Catheter tip
Needle

Cannula tip
Giving set spike

Injectable port
Rubber bung on drug containers

Key principles of ANTT

Always wash hands effectively

Never touch key parts/key sites

Touch non-key parts with confidence

Take appropriate infection control precautions

Aseptic non-touch technique overview

The Health and Social Care Act 2008: Code of Practice for the Prevention and Control of Healthcare Associated Infections has given rise to a number of clinical protocols that NHS bodies must adhere to. As a direct result of this, the aseptic non-touch technique (ANTT) has been instigated by many NHS Trusts.

The National Audit Office provide statistics regarding the number of patients who come to harm unnecessarily in the UK from hospital-acquired infection (HAI). Many people become infected during simple procedures, such as wound care, administration of intravenous medication and care of indwelling catheters, for example. Following investigation of these cases, root cause analysis often leads back to poor hand washing, poor cannula management and a failure to comply with correct procedures.

With a rise in MRSA bacteraemias, strategies to deliver on infection control targets were introduced. ANTT has developed considerably over the last 60 years, and, as a result, is now a safe, modern and efficient evidence-based aseptic technique. The standardization of this technique for clinical procedures aims to help reduce the risk of patients developing a HAI.

What is ANTT?

ANTT aims to prevent microorganisms from our hands, surfaces or equipment being introduced into an entry site for infection, by identification and protection of key parts of any procedure.

As practitioners, we need to ensure the treatment and procedures we carry out do not result in harm to our patients, and therefore ANTT must be used for all clinical procedures that by-pass the body's natural defences.

The principles of ANTT are simple:
- Always wash hands effectively (see Chapter 60, Hand washing, for the steps to follow).
- Never touch key parts/key sites.
- Touch non-key parts with confidence.
- Take appropriate infection control precautions.

The principle is that you cannot infect a key part if you don't touch it. By definition, a key part is a part of equipment or the site on a patient that, if contaminated with microorganisms, increases the risk of infection. The very tools that we use to perform health care are covered in bacteria, therefore maintaining ANTT means we need to adopt a robust hand-washing technique. Correct hand hygiene principles are the key to reducing HAI.

Key parts

Key sites include open wounds, insertion sites (cannula) and puncture sites (injections).

Infection control precautions

Appropriate infection control precautions need to be taken when carrying out ANTT procedures. Before the procedure is carried out, it is up to the health care professional to complete an assessment of the procedure in order to decide which precautions are required. Personal protective equipment such as gloves and aprons must be worn if there is a risk of exposure to or splashing/ spillage of body fluids.

Sterile versus non-sterile gloves often cause discussion. If it is possible to complete the procedure without touching key parts or key sites, then non-sterile gloves can be used. If it is deemed not possible, then sterile gloves must be used.

Following any clinical procedure, gloves and other personal protective equipment must be removed and disposed of appropriately following infection control and health and safety guidelines.

Non-sterile glove usage

Non-sterile gloves must be used for:
- intravenous medication administration
- venepuncture
- cannulation and removal of cannulas
- injection administration

Sterile glove usage

Sterile gloves must be used for:
- urinary catheterization
- central venous line insertion
- wound dressings

Clean working environment

Sterile towels and dressing packs are not always required, however, a clean working environment is a sensible precaution. The ideal environment for ANTT procedures is a designated clinic room if possible. If it is not possible and needs to be done at the patient's bedside, then it is advisable not to do it directly after bed making, as this will contribute to airborne contamination. In the community setting, careful consideration will need to be completed before starting the procedure. In all environments, windows must be closed and the use of electrical fans discouraged.

Cleaning of trays and surfaces must be completed with a sanitizing wipe to eliminate bacteria and microorganisms. More importantly, the surface needs adequate time to dry, otherwise it is not aseptic.

Roles and responsibilities

When a patient accesses health care, they have a right to be protected from preventable infections. Health care professionals have a duty to safeguard the well-being of patients when they are most vulnerable. While it is difficult to maintain sterility, it is important to reduce the risk of contamination.

In order to standardize practice, compliance is vital. It is therefore essential that health care professionals follow local guidelines and policies and are suitably educated in ANTT before carrying out any procedure.

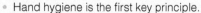

Key points
- Hand hygiene is the first key principle.
- Protect key parts or key sites at all times during the procedure, ensuring a non-touch technique.
- Follow local guidelines and policy with regards to cleaning key parts and key sites (such as medication bung, intravenous access port and skin preparations).
- Dispose of equipment and personal protective clothing according to infection control policy and health and safety guidelines.

62 Obtaining blood samples

Blood sampling in an infant, the dorsum of the hand is often the preferred site

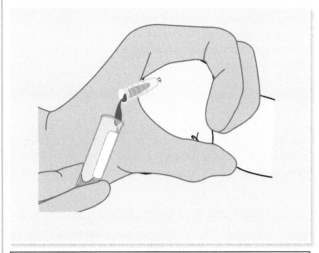

Sites for heel prick blood sample

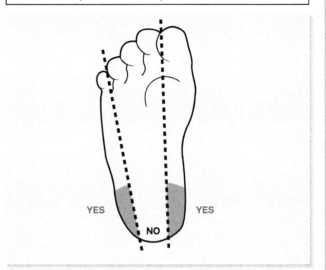

YES   NO   YES

Paediatric blood sample tubes

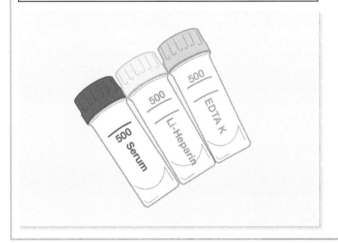

Obtaining blood samples overview

Venepuncture requires the introduction of a needle into a vein for the purposes of obtaining a blood sample for haematological, biochemical or bacteriological analysis. It can be traumatic for the child and family so careful preparation and planning are required.

This is one of the most common invasive procedures that is performed in clinical practice and is an essential component of clinical care that informs clinical decision-making. For the nurse who is performing venepuncture, it is their responsibility to be familiar with blood tests commonly undertaken, the requirements for each test (fasting, pre-drug administration), and know the normal blood component values.

Preparation of the child and family is key and needs to include the following elements:
• Explanation and rationale of the procedure and need to take blood.

• Previous history of venepuncture is useful to know.
• Informed consent.
• Involvement of play and distraction techniques.
• Analgesia, both local and systemic.

Principles

• The smallest gauge needle should be used in order to minimize damage to the vein. The vacuum system is likely to cause small veins to collapse so is not recommended for small children.
• If the child is receiving intravenous fluids, ideally another limb should be used but if this is not possible, then a vein below the level of the cannula should be chosen with the intravenous infusion stopped for 5–10 minutes prior to venepuncture.
• Avoid areas where a pulse is present as it is not desirable to accidently puncture an artery.
• Avoid areas where the skin is broken or where rashes are present.

Children and Young People's Nursing Skills at a Glance, First Edition. Edited by Elizabeth Gormley-Fleming and Deborah Martin.
© 2018 John Wiley & Sons, Ltd. Published 2018 by John Wiley & Sons, Ltd.

- Good infection control practice is essential.
- The age of the child will determine how the sample is drawn and the needle device used.
- On the blood sample tubes, identify the child by checking the name band and complete the information required on the blood sample tubes: name, hospital identification number, date of birth, sex, date and time sample taken.

Selection of a vein

Selecting the right vein is a very important aspect of venepuncture:
- The superficial veins of the arm are usually the site of choice in the child, namely, branches of the basilic, cephalic, median cephalic and median cubital vein.
- Care must always be taken to avoid the brachial artery and this should be done by palpation and then avoiding it.
- The vein should feel soft and bouncy, be straight and free from valves.
- In the infant, it may be difficult to palpate a vein so transillumination, i.e. the transmission of light through a sample, may be used.
- In the infant, the superficial veins in the dorsum of the hand, the dorsal venous arch or the metacarpal veins may be more accessible.
- Listen to the child, children who have blood taken on a regular basis will usually instruct you on which vein to use.
- The veins in the lower limbs should be avoided if at all possible, as the risk of thromboembolism has been identified.

Equipment

- Butterfly needle or needle-appropriate gauge: 25 or 23 gauge.
- Syringes.
- Vacuum system may be used in an older child.
- Disposable tourniquet.
- Alcohol swab.
- Appropriate collection tubes.
- Specimen request form.
- Low linting swab.
- Hypoallergenic plaster.
- Apron.
- Non-sterile gloves.
- Sharps bin.
- Light.

Procedure

- Wash and dry hands thoroughly.
- Apply non-sterile gloves and apron.
- Remove local anaesthetic cream.
- Bring the prepared equipment to the child.
- Assess veins and identify suitable vein/veins by palpation.
- Support limb with a pillow and ask parent/carer to hold child securely, ensuring that they are comfortable doing this and that child will be safe during the procedure. The child may wish to lie down.
- Apply tourniquet or ask staff to squeeze the limb being used gently. The older child could be asked to make a fist. The vein may be gently tapped or stroked in order to increase its prominence.
- Release the tourniquet.
- Wash and dry hands thoroughly.
- Apply non-sterile gloves and apron.
- Reapply the tourniquet.
- Clean skin with an alcohol-based solution for 30–60 seconds and allow to dry.
- Apply ethyl chloride spray if indicated as per manufacturer's instructions if topical anaesthetic cream has not been used.
- Remove the protective cover from the needle and inspect.
- Stabilize the skin with the thumb, stretching the skin downwards, or the vein can be stretched using the forefinger and thumb of the non-dominant hand. This will apply traction to the vein, thus anchoring it and preventing it rolling.
- Insert the needle at a 30° angle.
- Reduce the angle of descent when a flashback is seen. This will be in the tubing if using a butterfly device or in the hub of the needle if using a syringe. If using a syringe, pull back on the plunger of the syringe before commencing so that blood will flow into the syringe once the vein has been punctured.
- Slightly advance the needle into vein.
- Using very gentle pressure, withdraw the required amount of blood into the syringe. If using a needle, allow the blood to drip into the appropriate sample bottles without exerting any pressure on the needle.
- Loosen and remove tourniquet or relax pressure on limb.
- Remove needle from vein.
- Apply gentle digital pressure with the low lint swab over the puncture site for approximately one minute.
- Transfer the blood to the appropriate sample tubes in the correct order as soon as possible. Gently invert the tubes at least six times.
- Label all samples immediately.
- Inspect puncture site and apply sterile hypoallergenic plaster, checking their allergic status to plasters first.
- Ascertain comfort status of child.
- Dispose of all waste appropriately.
- Wash and dry hands.
- Document venepuncture in child's care records.

Heel or finger prick

Heel or finger pricking is not considered venepuncture as direct entry to a vein is not required.

It is important that when either of these sites are used, the correct area is identified and cleaned prior to piercing of the skin. Piercing of the skin is either with a barrelled needle or a lancing device. Blood flows freely through the needle into a specimen bottle, tube or directly onto collection paper (newborn blood spot screening). The same procedure as above should be followed once the appropriate sample has been obtained.

Key points
- Avoid tapping the vein, it does not make it more pronounced.
- Remove local anaesthetic cream within the prescribed timeframe to avoid local reactions.

63 Transfusion of blood and blood components

Unit of blood

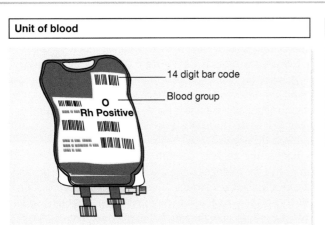

14 digit bar code

Blood group

O
Rh Positive

ABO blood group

Blood group	Antigen	Antibodies	Can donate to	Can receive blood from
A	Antigen A	Anti-B	A, AB	A, O
B	Antigen B	Anti-A	B, AB	B, O
AB	Antigen A Antigen B	NONE	AB	A, B, AB
O	NONE	Anti-A, Anti-B	A, B, AB, O	O

Blood transfusion reaction

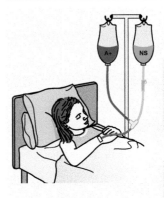

A+   NS

Febrile reaction:
Flushed appearance
Tachycardia
Rigor
Headache

Haemolytic reaction:
Loin pain
Hypotension
Haematuria
Pyrexia
Rigor
Tachycardia
Chest pain
Bronchospasm

Mild allergic reaction:
Urticaria
Pyrexia
Facial flushing

Immediate nursing care:

STOP transfusion and seek medical review of child

Serum sample tubes and cross-matching

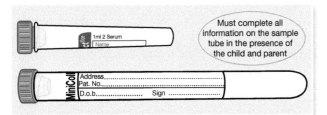

1ml 2 Serum
Name

Must complete all information on the sample tube in the presence of the child and parent

MiniColl
Address.................................
Pat. No.................................
D.o.b...................   Sign ....

Haemolytic disease of the newborn

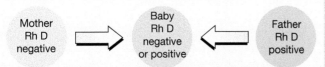

Mother Rh D negative → Baby Rh D negative or positive ← Father Rh D positive

Length of time for transfusion of blood and blood component

Blood/blood component	Length of transfusion time
Red cells	2–3 hours
Platelets	30 minutes
Fresh frozen plasma	30 minutes

Five points of bedside check

1 Ask the child to state their name and date of birth, let the child do this if able to do so.
2 Check identification of component against the infant's or child's wristband.
3 Check the prescription: has this component been prescribed?
4 Check the prescription: is this the correct component?
5 Check for specific requirements: does the patient need irradiated components or specially selected units?

Nursing implications:

- Stop transfusion and contact doctor
- Perform systematic assessment, A, B, C
- Treat symptoms; oxygen, intravenous anti-histamines and hydrocortisone as prescribed. Commence intravenous fluids as prescribed
- Obtain urine sample and check for presence of microscopic blood
- Assist with blood sampling
- Return unit of blood to transfusion laboratory with cross-match record forms
- Monitor child's vital signs

Children and Young People's Nursing Skills at a Glance, First Edition. Edited by Elizabeth Gormley-Fleming and Deborah Martin.
© 2018 John Wiley & Sons, Ltd. Published 2018 by John Wiley & Sons, Ltd.

Transfusion of blood and blood components overview

The safe transfusion of blood and blood products is an essential skill in everyday practice. The risk associated with this has the potential to be significant in terms of harm to the infant or child. Transfusion-transmitted infections are a potential hazard. A complex procedure, a safe transfusion practice depends on good teamwork at every stage of this multi-faceted procedure. In accordance with the Blood Safety and Quality Regulation (2005), it is a legal requirement that every unit of blood is traceable from donor to recipient.

Why transfuse?

Infants and children generally require red cell transfusion to treat anaemia and haemorrhage. Diagnosis of anaemia is confirmed by measurement of haemoglobin levels. There is no threshold level for transfusion; a complete clinical assessment will determine the need to transfuse with red cells.

Platelets and fresh frozen plasma may be administered when thrombocytopenia is diagnosed to prevent or to cease haemorrhage.

Blood groups

There are over 200 identified blood groups, however, it is the ABO and Rh D blood systems that are familiar to nursing practice. Blood groups are inherited. The ABO group is identified in the table. Patients with blood group A will have an A antigen on the membrane of their red cells. Its function is to stimulate the production of anti-B antibodies that circulate in the plasma and offer defence to the body against B antigens that are present on the surface of the red cell membrane of B and AB red cells. Thus, a patient who is blood group A can only receive group A or group O blood, as people who are blood group O have neither A or B antigens and they produce A and B antibodies in their plasma.

Rh D refers to its presence or absence on the surface of the red cell membrane. When present, the patient will be Rh D positive, when absent, it will be reported as Rh D negative blood group. Antibodies against the Rh factor are developed through placental sensitization or transfusion. Haemolytic disease of the newborn may occur when the mother is Rh D negative and the biological father is Rh D positive and the baby's blood is Rh D positive. When the baby's blood crosses into the mother's circulation via the placenta, Rh D antibodies may be produced by her immune system, resulting in haemolysis of the baby's red cells.

Transfusion procedure

Pre-transfusion

The first step in the transfusion procedure is to obtain a blood sample from the child for a group and save it. This must be done for each blood transfusion required. The identity of the infant/child must be ascertained and consent given along with relevant information. When a cross-match is required, the date, time and number of units or volume (for infants) required must be identified on the request form. The request form and blood sample must have the patient's first name, surname, date of birth, NHS or hospital number, and gender, and be signed and dated by the person drawing the blood sample before leaving the infant's/child's bedside and before the sample is sent to the laboratory. Local policy must be adhered to at all stages of the blood/blood product administration procedure.

Preparing the child for a transfusion

• Ensure consent is obtained and the procedure understood by the child and parents/carers with potential problems made aware to them as they will need to alert healthcare staff promptly if any such problems occur.
• Assist with the cannulation procedure in accordance with local guidelines, ensuring the cannula is secured correctly and is patent by flushing it using a pulsatile flushing action with 0.9% sodium chloride.
• Pre-transfusion medication should be administered as prescribed.
• Ensure the blood or blood product has been prescribed on the infant's/child's prescription chart with the name of the blood component/product to be administered clearly legible, the amount to be transfused and the duration of transfusion stated.
• Record the temperature, heart rate/pulse, respiratory rate, blood pressure and SaO_2 level as a baseline and note these as pre-transfusion observations on the infant's/child's chart.
• Arrange for the blood component to be collected giving the four points of patient identification to the person designated to collect it:
  1 Forename
  2 Surname
  3 Date of birth
  4 Hospital identification/NHS number.

Receipt of blood component

The collection document must be signed, ideally by the health care professional who requested it, and it should have the four points of patient identification, the time of collection and the time of delivery. The blood component should be checked and the transfusion commenced immediately or as soon as possible on its receipt in the clinical area. If delayed, then the blood transfusion laboratory must be contacted for advice.

The administration of blood/blood products

• Before commencing the transfusion, a final bedside check must be done. The 14-digit donation number on the National Blood Service unit label bar code should match the unit identification label on the compatibility tag attached to the bag.
• Check the patient information on the unit with the infant's/child's identification wristband: they should match.
• Prime the intravenous administration giving set with the blood/blood product. The type of giving set to be used will depend on the product being administered. Commence the infusion at the prescribed rate. The rate of the infusion will depend on the product being administered. When transfusing red cells, the rate of the infusion should be slower for the first 15 minutes than the prescribed rate. In an emergency situation, transfusion rates may be increased.

Care of the child during the transfusion

• Complete the set of baseline observations.
• After 15 minutes, a repeat set of observations must be recorded. Ideally the nurse should remain with the child for the first 15 minutes of the transfusion as the majority of reactions occur during this period.
• A complete set of observations must be recorded at the end of the transfusion of each unit. If subsequent units are to be transfused, this forms the baseline for their administration.
• The clinical condition of the infant/child will determine the frequency of vital sign measurements. Local policy must be adhered to.

- Frequent visual checks are important and any reported concerns of the parents must be listened to and appropriate action taken.
- Administer any prescribed transfusion-related medication as per the medication chart, e.g. furosemide.

Points to note when transfusing platelets

- Administer platelets prior to a red cell transfusion.
- Never store platelets in a refrigerator.
- Use a platelet administration set.
- Agitate before administration.
- As platelets are transfused rapidly, visual observation of the infant/child is important to note adverse reactions.

Points to note when transfusing fresh frozen plasma

- Administer prior to a red cells transfusion.
- Return to blood transfusion laboratory if not going to be administered within 30 minutes of receipt in clinical area.
- Use a blood component administration set.
- As fresh frozen plasms (FFP) is transfused rapidly, visual observation of the infant/child is important to note adverse reactions.

Points to note when transfusing red cells

- Contact blood transfusion laboratory if not administered within 30 minutes of receipt in clinical area.
- Transfuse using a sterile blood component administration set with a 170–200 υm filter.
- Remain with patient for first 15 minutes during which time the transfusion should be at a slower rate than that prescribed.
- Must only be administered to the patient who is named on the compatibility tag.

End of transfusion

- All empty units must remain in the clinical area until the current transfusion is completed and then returned to the blood transfusion laboratory or disposed of in the clinical area as per local policy dictates.
- If the child has had an adverse reaction, then the bag must be returned to the blood transfusion laboratory.
- Ensure the transfusion procedure has been documented accurately in the infant's/child's records.

Adverse reactions

Adverse reactions range from mild to severe. They can be life-threatening and are mostly due to ABO incompatibility as a result of human error or misidentification of the infant/child at any stage in the transfusion process.

Mild reaction

- Increase in temperature of 1.5° above the infant's/child's baseline. Usually mild reactions occur within the first 15 minutes.
- The infant/child should be checked for the presence of an urticarial rash.

Moderate to severe

The following effects may appear:

- feeling dizzy;
- loss of consciousness;
- wheeze;
- bronchospasm;
- loin pain;
- abdominal pain;
- breathlessness;
- pyrexia;
- tachycardia;
- tremors;
- urticaria;
- haematuria.

Infective shock

Symptoms of infective shock are:

- muscle pain;
- pyrexia;
- hypotension;
- tachycardia;
- rigors;
- wheeze/dyspnoea;
- shocked appearance.

Irrespective of the nature of the reaction, the transfusion MUST always be stopped immediately and prompt medical review must occur. If the child has collapsed, then begin basic life support.

Key points

- Transfusion at night should be avoided unless clinical need indicates otherwise.
- The final bedside check where the component to be administered is checked against the child's prescription chart and their identification is essential to avoid error.
- Blood components to be administered to children should be in volume based on their weight but must never exceed the standard accepted dose that an adult would receive.

64 Cannulation

Sites for cannulation

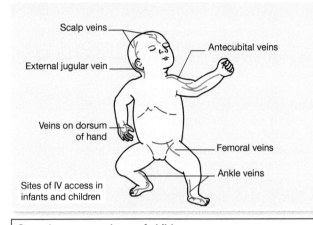

Sites of IV access in infants and children

Cannula and named parts

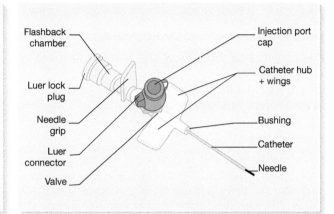

Cannula gauge and age of child

Cannula gauge size	Age of child
26	Neonate and infant
24	Child
22	Older child
18	Older child in an emergency situation

Cannula in situ in vein

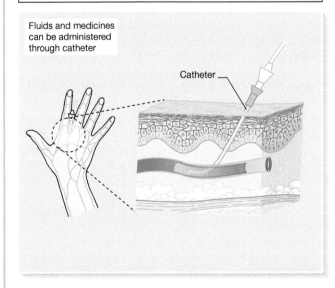

Fluids and medicines can be administered through catheter

Catheter

Transparent dressing in situ

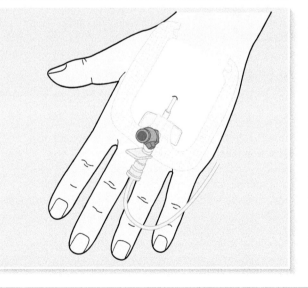

Children and Young People's Nursing Skills at a Glance, First Edition. Edited by Elizabeth Gormley-Fleming and Deborah Martin.
© 2018 John Wiley & Sons, Ltd. Published 2018 by John Wiley & Sons, Ltd.

Cannulation overview

Peripheral intravenous cannulae are increasingly being inserted by nurses and this is considered to be an extended role. This involves the insertion of a flexible plastic tube into a vein, thus providing direct access to the circulatory system for the purpose of administration of intravenous fluids and medication.

Indications for use

- Short-term therapy: 3–5 days.
- Bolus injections or short intermittent infusions.

Choice of device

The principle of using the smallest, shortest gauge cannula in any given situation should be adhered to.

Insertion site

This will depend on the age of the child, the clinical condition, and indication for use, type and duration of therapy and the condition of the child's veins. Previous history of infusion devices should be considered. The antecubital fossas (median vein), the dorsum of hands (dorsal venous network) and wrists are common sites for the insertion of a cannula in a child. The scalp and long saphenous vein of the lower limb may also be used in infants if none of the other areas are suitable. In an older child, the basilica vein or cephalic vein may also be used. Where possible, areas of flexion should be avoided and the child should be given a choice about the site used. Areas where skin is broken or inflamed should also be avoided.

Choosing a vein

The vein to be cannulated should be selected and should be easy to palpate, feel bouncy, refill when depressed, be straight and free from valves. Valves may be felt as small lumps and the presence of valves will make it difficult to advance the cannula and to get backflow of blood.

Procedure

Prior to insertion of the cannula, the following points should be considered:
- Gain consent from the child and/or parents.
- Check the child's identity and review the treatment plan.
- Distraction therapy organized.
- Correct use of local anaesthetic topical agents.
- Use of sucrose for the young infant (Stevens et al. 2003).
- Familiarization with correct holding technique for procedure (RCN 2003).
- Assess veins for suitability.
- Follow local NHS Trust's policy for insertion of cannula.
- Competence in Aseptic Non-Touch Technique (ANTT) (see Chapter 61).

Equipment

- Cannulae of the appropriate gauge.
- Tissues to remove local anaesthetic cream.
- Skin cleansing solution.
- Extension set with smartsite.
- 0.9% normal saline drawn up into 10 ml syringe.
- Ethyl chloride spray.
- Entonox (if it is going to be used).
- Specimen bottles if sample to be collected at the same time.
- Non-sterile gloves.
- Cottonwool balls.
- Tourniquet, disposable.
- Sterile dressing.
- Splint.
- Kling bandage.
- Non-sterile tape.
- Portable light.

Procedure

- Assess the child and family and their level of understanding once you have given them a full explanation of the procedure. Consent should be obtained at this point.
- Assemble the required team members: a nurse to hold the limb, a play therapist/nurse to distract the child.
- Ensure privacy for the child.
- Check all the equipment is ready.
- Wash and dry hands thoroughly.
- If child's skin is visibly dirty, then this should be washed with soapy water and dried.
- Remove local anaesthetic cream.
- Assess veins and identify suitable vein/veins by palpation.
- Wash and dry hands thoroughly again.
- Apply non-sterile gloves and apron.
- Support limb with a pillow and ask parent/carer to hold child securely, ensuring that they are comfortable doing this and that child will be safe during the procedure.
- Apply a tourniquet or ask staff to squeeze the limb being used gently.
- Clean skin with an alcohol-based solution for 30–60 seconds and allow it to dry.
- Apply ethyl chloride spray if indicated as per manufacturer's instructions.
- Remove needle guard and check the cannula
- Stabilize the skin with the thumb, stretching the skin downwards, or the vein can be stretched using the forefinger and thumb of the non-dominant hand. This will apply traction to the vein, thus anchoring it and preventing it rolling.
- Hold cannula with bevelled end up, enter skin at 10–45° angle (Dougherty and Lister 2008) and using a steady motion, advance cannula until a 'flashback' of blood is seen in the chamber of the cannula.
- Decrease the angle of the cannula so as to prevent puncture of the posterior vein wall and gently advance the cannula off the stylet. Continue to insert the plastic cannula into the vein while keeping the skin taut until the hub of the cannula is touching the skin.
- Never re-introduce the stylet into the plastic cannula once you have removed it.
- Loosen and remove the tourniquet or relax pressure on limb.
- Apply pressure with one finger to the vein above the insertion site and fully remove the stylet.
- Secure the cannula with an appropriate transparent sterile dressing such as Tagederm IV™.
- If blood samples are to be obtained, do so now before flushing the cannula. Attach an extension set to the cannula with a 10 ml syringe and withdraw the required amount of blood. Gentle squeezing pressure or a tourniquet may need to be used again at this stage.
- Attach the extension tubing with the smartsite in situ, and using a 10 ml syringe primed with 0.9% normal saline, flush the cannula using a pulsatile flush, ending with positive pressure and close the clamp.

- Inspect the site for signs of leakage or swelling and clean away any blood from area.
- Apply the correct size disposable splint and cover with a bandage.
- Ensure the child and parent/carer are comfortable and pain-free. Explain altered care needs, i.e. restriction in movement now that cannula is inserted.
- Remove gloves, wash hands and dispose of all waste correctly, following universal precautions.
- Document insertion in care records and place intravenous cannula care bundle in child's care records.

Cannula care

When a cannula has been inserted, a cannula care plan should be completed and signed with the date and time the cannula was inserted. Whenever the cannula needs to be accessed, all bandaging and supportive dressing should be removed so that the cannula site can be visually inspected. This assessment should be documented on the care plan. A visual infusion phlebitis (VIP) score should be used.

When to remove a cannula

A cannula should be removed in the following cases:
- If there is extravasation and infiltration.
- If intravenous access is no longer required.
- It may no longer be functioning effectively.
- It may be causing the child excessive discomfort.

How to remove a cannula

The child can be actively involved in removing the dressing covering the cannula if they want. First, remove all dressings, gently put pressure over the cannula site with an appropriate dressing. Remove the cannula gently and apply pressure until the bleeding has stopped, then cover with an appropriate dressing. Ensure the cannula removed is intact prior to disposal. Dispose of as per local policy.

Key points
- Analgesia should be administered systemically and topically prior to insertion.
- Use play therapy and distraction techniques.
- Visual inspection of the insertion site is essential to identify and prevent phlebitis.
- Local policy must be adhered to.

References

Dougherty, L. and Lister, S. (2008) *The Royal Marsden Hospital Manual of Clinical Nursing Procedures*. Wiley Blackwell, Oxford.
RCN (Royal College of Nursing) (2003) *Children and Young People's Nursing: A Philosophy of Care. Guidance for Nursing Staff*. RCN, London.
Stevens B., McGrath, P., Gibbins, S. et al. (2003) Procedural pain in newborns at risk for neurologic impairment. *Pain* 105(1–2): 27–35.

65 Care of the dying child

Barriers to effective communication in end-of-life care
Source: Together for Short Lives (2012) A guide to end of life care

- Fear of making things worse or not being able to answer difficult questions

- Lack of confidence in starting conversations exploring concerns or closing conversations

- Workplace issues such as environment, workload priorities, lack of support or training

Common symptoms at end of life

- Seizures/convulsions
- Pain
- Vomiting
- Agitation
- Fatigue
- Constipation
- Poor appetite
- Sadness/depression
- Excessive secretions

Deaths by age group, as percentage of total, UK
Source: Office for National Statistics (2012)

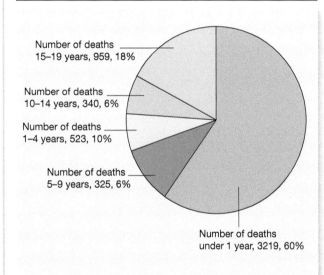

Number of deaths 15–19 years, 959, 18%
Number of deaths 10–14 years, 340, 6%
Number of deaths 1–4 years, 523, 10%
Number of deaths 5–9 years, 325, 6%
Number of deaths under 1 year, 3219, 60%

Key people involved in end-of-life care

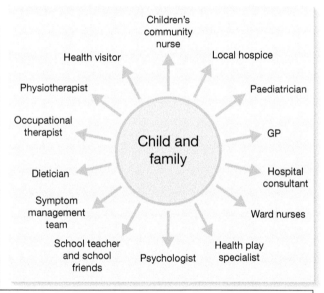

Children's community nurse
Health visitor
Local hospice
Physiotherapist
Paediatrician
Occupational therapist
GP
Child and family
Dietician
Hospital consultant
Symptom management team
Ward nurses
School teacher and school friends
Psychologist
Health play specialist

Points of note

- *Good communication will enhance the experience of end-of-life care for families and the child. Sensitivity and compassion should be demonstrated throughout the process*

- *Children have a right to be involved in their care. Care planning, wherever appropriate, should respect the child's wishes and choices*

- *Symptom management planning is key to maintaining a quality of life for the child and maintaining their dignity. Symptom management plans should be regularly evaluated and updated*

- *Care should be taken to communicate honestly with the family when choosing the child's place of death, giving them all the options and reassuring them that they can change their mind if they feel this is necessary*

Children and Young People's Nursing Skills at a Glance, First Edition. Edited by Elizabeth Gormley-Fleming and Deborah Martin.
© 2018 John Wiley & Sons, Ltd. Published 2018 by John Wiley & Sons, Ltd.

Care of the dying child overview

In the United Kingdom in 2012, over 5000 children under the age of 19 died. This is illustrated per age group in the figure opposite, demonstrating that children under 1 year make up over half of the deaths in the UK for those under 19. Late adolescence (15–19 years old) makes up the second biggest group. There are varying reasons why children die in childhood and while some deaths can be planned with the child and family, other deaths can be very sudden. The nurse plays a key role in caring for the dying child and there are many elements that can contribute to effective support for a child and family.

Communication

Communication is an essential component of end-of-life care and the literature frequently highlights the skills required for effective communication. Breaking bad news or having difficult conversations can be hard for all medical professionals but the aim of good communication is to ensure the family and child are continuously involved and understand what is being said to them. Sensitivity and compassion are key to achieving good communication but nurses must be aware of barriers that may arise when delivering end-of-life care. The United Kingdom has a diverse range of religions and cultures. Therefore, an appreciation and understanding of a child and family's beliefs must be acknowledged early on when planning for end of life. Health care professionals should uphold the wishes and beliefs of the family at all times and open communication will help to achieve this. It is also important to note that there are variations of faith and thus conversations to explore a family's individual cultural and spiritual needs should take place.

Involving children

Article 12 of the United Nations Convention on the Rights of the Child requires involvement of the dying child in the decision-making process. Some children may be too young to understand exactly what is happening, however, they will still be able to have a say in their care and literature has demonstrated that children as young as 4 can provide insights into health experiences. With effective communication, nurses can work with parents to establish the best way to involve children in the decision-making process and can be a key advocate for the child and family. Involving children at the end of life can ensure that holistic care takes place and physical, emotional and spiritual needs are met. Some children at the end of life may want to discuss things without their parents present and, where possible, this should be facilitated. Some hospices have programmes to enable this to happen, as well as sibling support services which are also an important part in caring for the whole family.

Symptom management planning

Symptom management is a large part of end-of-life care, with the main aim being to maintain a quality of life for the child and ensure their comfort. Some of the most commonly reported symptoms at the end of life are highlighted in the figure opposite. An individual symptom management care plan should be written in conjunction with the child and family and this should be regularly evaluated and updated. Depending on the child's condition, evaluation may take place weekly, daily or even hourly. For example, a child who is still tolerating oral medication may become unconscious and therefore another route of medication may be required. Parents should be given details of who to contact if they are worried/anxious/have any questions or if they feel their child needs further symptom management. In the hospital and hospice setting, a nurse is readily available for parents to consult, in the community setting it is important for parents to have up-to-date contact numbers, including numbers for out of hours service provision. Non-pharmacological methods of symptom management should always be discussed and professionals such as health play specialists or psychologists may be a good resource to support this.

Place of death

Increasingly children are able to die at home with their family around them. Just because this may be a viable option, however, it should not be assumed that this is what the family wants or would choose. When caring for a dying child, it may be that a child is moved from one setting to another. This can mean that there are many professionals involved in the child's care, just how many people may be involved in the figure opposite. Communication and joined-up working must therefore be a priority for all professionals and it may be wise to appoint a key professional or service to facilitate a child's care. It is important to ensure that families have all the information available to them and understand the benefits and disadvantages of each setting. Professionals should also be aware of local policies and procedures to be followed following a child's death in different settings.

Key points
- Children are often aware that they are dying and may ask questions that may not have answers.
- All family members should be involved as much or as little as they wish.
- Bereavement counselling should be offered.

References

Office for National Statistics (2012) Available at: https: www.ons.gov .uk
Together for Short Lives (2012) *A Guide to End of Life Care*. Together for Short Lives, Bristol.

66 Care after death

Useful resources

- Together for Short Lives, (2012) *The Verification of Expected Death in Childhood: Guidance for Children's Palliative Care Services*
- The Child Bereavement Network www.childhoodbereavementnetwork.org.uk
- Dying Matters Coalition www.dyingmatters.org
- Multi-faith index www.mfghc.com
- Together for Short Lives http://www.togetherforshortlives.org.uk/

Procedures for unexpected deaths

Rapid Response Process – this involves a group of specialist key professionals who respond to the unexpected death of a child. They investigate and evaluate each death, piecing together key information

Coroner – judicial officer who investigates death in certain circumstances. This person is usually a doctor or lawyer with more than 5 years experience

Post-mortem – involves examining organs and tissue to identify possible conditions that may have caused death. By law, a post-mortem is required for any sudden death where the cause is unknown. Parents and medical professionals can also request a post-mortem to establish cause of death

Supporting staff

- Regular training should be provided in order that best practice and up-to-date information are shared
- Enhanced training in communication may be beneficial for staff
- Opportunities for junior staff to shadow more experienced staff should be provided
- Good relationships with other agencies such as hospices should be encouraged. This enables inter-disciplinary support and learning
- Debriefs should be available following the death of a child in a setting
- Counselling or further support opportunities should be available and offered to staff where required

Considerations when deciding where a child's body is kept prior to the funeral

At home
- Radiators must be turned off, but this may not be practical in winter months
- Cooling unit will be necessary, this cannot always be guaranteed as another family may be using it
- Deterioration of the body may mean it is not practical for the body to stay at home after a certain period of time
- Some siblings may find it scary for a dead body to be in the house

Hospice cool room
- Hospices generally only have one cool room and this can only be used if free
- This may not be an option to all families if the child has not met the criteria for the hospice prior to death
- The hospice may be a long drive from the family home, and if the family are not staying at the hospice, it can make them feel a long way from their child

Funeral directors
- No option to stay with the child's body
- Times for visiting may be restricted
- Some funeral directors will charge for viewing of the body to take place

Physical changes to a dead body

Changes to the eyes – if the eyelids are not closed before or very shortly after death, they can be very difficult to close. Some families find this distressing. Advice should be sought from the undertaker.

Livor mortis – this is the discoloration of the skin due to pooling of the blood after circulation stops. It occurs within half an hour of death and becomes 'fixed' after about 10–12 hours. For a child lying on their back after death, the blood will pool on their buttocks, their back and the back of their legs and head.

Leaking of body fluids – leakage is common but can be further heightened, depending on the condition the child had before they died. Urinary and faecal leakage are common and pads can be placed under the child to deal with this. On moving the child, leakage from the mouth or nose can also occur and suction, wet wipes and/or flannels can be used to deal with this.

Rigor mortis – this is the stiffening of muscles, which can become apparent within 3–4 hours of death. This is important to explain to parents when they are requesting their child be dressed in a particular outfit. Rigor mortis disappears 36–48 hours after death.

Points of note

- There are certain procedures and policies that must be followed after the death of the child. These will differ depending on whether death was expected or unexpected

- Health care professionals can support the family to carry out personal care after death, they can also support the family to understand the physical changes that happen to a dead body

- There are many helpful resources that can be used to signpost families to further post-bereavement and support groups. Professionals should keep up to date in the knowledge of what is locally available for families

- Staff should be adequately supported throughout end-of-life care and care after death. Further training and opportunities for shadowing should be provided

Children and Young People's Nursing Skills at a Glance, First Edition. Edited by Elizabeth Gormley-Fleming and Deborah Martin.
© 2018 John Wiley & Sons, Ltd. Published 2018 by John Wiley & Sons, Ltd.

Care after death overview

After a child dies, there are certain procedures and policies in place that must be followed. This must be done with great sensitivity and must respect the needs and wishes of each individual family. The procedures and policies to be followed are dependent on whether a child's death was expected or unexpected. This chapter will focus on care after an expected death but practitioners must also familiarize themselves with procedures in place for unexpected deaths.

Legal requirements after death

• *Verification* – This is confirmation that the child has died. This can be done by a nurse but can also be done by a medical practitioner or another registered professional who has been deemed competent to do so. It is focusing on the physiological assessment to confirm death, for example, observing for breathing for a good period of time, looking for signs of life and listening for a heartbeat. The family should be supported throughout.

• *Certification* – By law, a medical practitioner has to certify the cause of death. This is a statutory requirement. This is completed by the medical practitioner who was attending to the child or had seen them last. If the child has died at home, this will usually be completed by the child's General Practitioner. A 'Medical Certification of Cause of Death' must be completed, which involves:

  • a statement of the cause of death;
  • the date the child died;
  • the date the child was last seen alive;
  • whether they have seen the body after death.

• *Registration of death* – A Medical Certification of Cause of Death is required to register the death. The family can now legally dispose of the child's body. After registering the death, the family will receive a certified copy of the Death Certificate. This provides them with an explanation of the cause of death and why the child died. This is useful for their family's medical records.

Looking after the family

Caring for a grieving family can be incredibly challenging but it is a very important part of nursing care. Care should be taken to gently guide the family through the activities that need to be done at their own pace. Consideration, however, must be given to the condition of the body and health care professionals must balance this with meeting the needs of the family. It is anticipated that conversations will have taken place about care after death in the cases where death was expected, including where the child's body will be stored. Parents do not have to adhere to the original plan though, and some parents find that after death they want to deviate from the plan. This must not be discouraged and parents need to understand that whatever they choose is acceptable.

Care of the dead body

Following the verification of death, the family can be supported to carry out personal care to the child. The optimal time to do this is within two hours as rigor mortis will begin at this time. The limbs should be straightened out and medical devices such as cannulas, tracheostomies and gastrostomies should be removed as per local policy. No devices should be removed if a post mortem is required. Insertion sites and wounds should be cleaned and a dressing applied. If there is likely to be any exudate, the dressing should be waterproof. Jewellery should be removed unless the parents wish otherwise. Legible identity bands in accordance with local policy must be applied to the child's body. Some parents may want to be present, whereas others may find this too distressing. The nurse can also support families to wash and dress the child and many families appreciate the support in doing this. The child's body should then be covered with a clean sheet and a toy or flower placed with the child as the parent wish. Some physical changes may happen after death.

Storing the body after death

As part of advanced care planning, parents (sometimes in discussion with the child) may have decided where they want the body to be kept after death and before the funeral. Options that may be available to families are for the body to be kept at home, at a hospice or at the funeral directors. Not all options will be available to all families, however, and considerations of each option are outlined.

• *At home* – keeping a child's body at home may be the preferred option for some families at it means they continue to feel close to the child and family members can visit to say goodbye.

• *Hospice* – most hospices have a designated 'cool room' where the child's body can be kept after death and have an adjoining family suite where the family can stay also. Some families find it useful to have the support of hospice staff after a child's death and it has been found that parents who had used a hospice cool room reported feeling physically, practically and emotionally supported during this time.

• *Funeral directors* – a child's body can be stored here until the funeral. The funeral director will manage the condition of the body in a professional and sensitive way.

The grieving process

The death of a child has a profound impact on parents, siblings, grandparents and many more family members and friends. Each individual will grieve and express grief in their own way and this should be respected, but health care workers do have a role in the grieving process and there are certain protective factors that have been offered for 'successful bereavement'. These include the benefit of adequate information giving and pre-bereavement counselling. Health care professionals may offer signposting to other services to support the grieving process, although their purpose is not to show the family how to grieve, but to support them as necessary and with respect to individual spiritual, cultural and religious needs.

Supporting staff

Staff can be greatly affected following end-of-life care and care of the family following death.

Key points
• Accurate documentation is important.
• Explanations to the family at every stage are important.

Reference

Together for Short Lives (2012) *The Verification of Expected Death in Childhood: Guidance for Children's Palliative Care Service*. Together for Short Lives, Bristol.

Index

Children and Young People's Nursing Skills at a Glance, First Edition. Edited by Elizabeth Gormley-Fleming and Deborah Martin.
© 2018 John Wiley & Sons, Ltd. Published 2018 by John Wiley & Sons, Ltd.